HOMEOPATHY
AN ILLUSION

HOMEOPATHY
AN ILLUSION

Dinesh Kumar Jain
Associate Professor
Pharmacology Deptt.
G.R. Medical College, Gwalior (M.P.)

PEACOCK BOOKS

Published by
PEACOCK BOOKS
7/22, Ansari Road, Darya Ganj, New Delhi-110 002
Phones : 2327 3880, 2327 5880, 2328 0451
Fax : +91-11-2328 5873
E-mail : info@atlanticbooks.com
Web : www.atlanticbooks.com

Branch Office
5, Nallathambi Street, Wallajah Road,
Chennai-600 002
Phones : +91-44-6461 1085, 3241 3319
E-mail : chennai@atlanticbooks.com

Peacock Books is an imprint of
Atlantic Publishers and Distributors (P) Ltd.

ISBN 978-81-248-0195-6

Printed in India at Nice Printing Press, A-33/3A, Site-IV,
Industrial Area, Sahibabad, Ghaziabad, U.P.

FOREWORD

In questions of science the authority of a thousand is not worth the humble reasoning of a single individual.

This book which is a treasure trove of information regarding Homeopathic system of medicine is in real sense a humble reasoning of various unanswered questions and queries regarding its principles and scientific basis of its remedies. While making huge research on and assessment of Homeopathic principles and its other aspects the learned author, who is a renowned medical teacher, expert pharmacologist, psychiatrist, philosopher, and intellectual, chose rational and logical modern scientific approach purely to find truth. He is unbiased, non-judgemental and with an open mind questions irrationally held beliefs pertaining to Homeopathy that may be more harmful for the modern scientific principles and patients at large.

Samuel Hahnemann (1755-1843), a German Physician, formulated Homeopathy's basic principles in the late eighteenth century. In those days modern scientific medicine was in infancy. Now, after Hahnemann, the Homeopaths had over 150 years to demonstrate the effectiveness of their medicine and prove its basic principles but they miserably failed. This is an age of information and reasoning and it is a pity that we are still waiting for proof. Homeopathy is popular largely in ignorant people irrespective of their financial and educational status. Ignorance never settles questions. In this respect the author has done a commendable job to clear the cobwebs of ignorance surrounding Homeopathy and I hope that the readers, specially doctors and students of science, will be immensely benefited by this treatise.

The problem with present-day Homeopaths and self-acclaimed advocates of Homeopathy is that they are boasters and claim that Homeopathic medicines are a panacea and can treat any disease including cancer, diabetes and genetic diseases. If we see the history of modern medical science we will find that great men and great scientists have not been boasters but perceivers. This is a well known practice of modern medical science that it never boasts or advocates irrationally held beliefs or accepts any hypothesis on the basis of unproven flimsy facts.

Life of man is short and we make it still shorter by careless but fatal faith in Homeopathy. Presently, modern medical science asserts that Homeopathy is not a science and its remedies have been at most places, both effective and ineffective. Its subjective feeling of well-being in patients is explained by the fact that all diseases have some psychosomatic elements and on an average Homeopathic physicians give more time to their patients; it has significant calming effect and psychological pseudo-assurance of medical attention on patients, resulting into a feeling of well-being. In reality, several dangers are looming large on such patients particularly when they are suffering from some serious chronic diseases. Major danger of Homeopathic system of medicine is not due to direct harm but due to indirect damage. This is because of encouragement of self-diagnosis and treatment, recent trend of commercial use of unknown herbs and chemicals in the garb of Homeopathic remedies and most importantly undertreatment or rather no specific treatment alongwith Homeopathic remedies to those patients who are suffering from cancer, diabetes, hypertension and other serious chronic diseases. This results into severe complications, often even death. Most of such unfortunate end-stage patients finally find their way into allopathic hospitals and die or have serious complications beyond the scope of treatment by the modern medical system. This stimulates the ignorant people and their relatives to further blame the allopathic system for the pitiable condition or death of patients. This vicious cycle goes on and on and ironically, further enhances the popularity of Homeopathy as a harmless system of medicine, while the ultimate truth is that pseudo-confidence developed in patients after taking Homeopathic remedies and their subsequent carefree attitude are indirectly responsible for death or serious complications of these hapless patients.

Therefore, the effort of the author has become more relevant and significant for clearing the confusions and misconceptions regarding the myth of Homeopathy which has superstitiously acquired a place of alternative medical system without qualifying the painstaking acid tests of modern scientific methods. I hope the readers will be more knowledgeable after reading this book.

Bharat Jain
Professor and Head,
Department of Pathology
G.R. Medical College,
Gwalior (M.P.)

PREFACE

Nowadays, Ayurveda, Homeopathy, Yoga and other alternative systems of medicine are popular in India and many other parts of the world. People also take the help of astrology and religion for treatment. The Government of India is also supporting these systems of therapeutics which are unscientific, illogical, unreliable and not based on proper experimental work.

A conscientious medical student, having a professional approach and a genuine concern for the sick and ailing, can never promote Homeopathy. If various illogical and unscientific therapies are prevalent in the society, the specialists of modern medical science are only to be blamed. Actually, they never tried to explore the facts. If useless and unscientific therapeutic methods are being practised in the society, it is the responsibility of the medical fraternity to put facts before the people. If we get respect and recognition from the society, it is our most important and earnest duty to protect the society from the dangers being caused by the harmful practices of unscientific and useless therapeutic methods. Crores of rupees are being spent on alternative systems of medicine unnecessarily. Due to this, tuberculosis, leprosy, malaria and other curable diseases are spreading dangerously. Modern medical science is highly effective in these ailments but the use of alternative system of medicine makes them incurable and unbeatable. The medical community should take the responsibility to fight this menace. They should not keep silent but oppose this strongly. Only then we will be able to fulfill our duty as responsible citizens.

My acknowledgements are due to Dr. Ashok Kumar Jain, working in the Department of Pharmacology, G.R. Medical College, Gwalior, without whose precious help it would have been very difficult to accomplish this work. I record my deep sense of appreciation for his invaluable help and cooperation.

I am highly indebted to Professor P.R. Pandey and Dr. Deepak Johary for going through the manuscript, making suggestions and adding to my expression, in many ways.

My findings on the subject of Homeopathy have been published in the *Journal of Pharmacovigilance & Drug Safety.*

The book will be highly useful to the medical fraternity as well as the non-medical fraternity, i.e. common people, in dispelling several myths associated with Homeopathy. It will help them in developing a rational approach towards it based on scientific facts.

Dinesh Kumar Jain

INTRODUCTION

Superstition and development of knowledge are two contradictory concepts in a society. The concepts and beliefs that are prevalent in society, if genuine, based on logic and reason, need no reformation and thus would continue to be practised. But this does not hold true. Development of knowledge means collection and analysis of new information and addition of new knowledge. Thus, on the basis of evolved knowledge, change in the society is a normal practice of healthy community.

One of the most important aims of human life is to develop potential and do creative work for the welfare of the society and the new generation.

Knowledge is the collection of information. Intelligence is the capacity to analyse the information and discover the knowledge. Knowledge can be given or gained through the medium of education. Literacy is the knowledge of reading and writing.

Creation of knowledge is a continuous process. The history of knowledge is closely associated with the history of human beings. Continuous effort towards the growth of a civilization leads to continuous accumulation of knowledge.

In earlier times, there was limited knowledge. Today we have a vast ocean of knowledge, which is the sum of creative efforts of thousands of years of billions of human beings. The new generation has the knowledge of old generation. The new generation, by its intelligence and available resources further enriches its knowledge. In coming years, knowledge would be much larger than it was earlier. On the basis of this knowledge, new concepts and new thoughts can be deduced for the welfare of humanity. The new generation has greater knowledge than the older generation. That's why it can take more accurate decisions than the older generation and it can also change decisions and assumptions of the older generations.

Due to lack of knowledge even an intelligent person is unable take the right decision. There should be a proper coordination of intelligence and knowledge to reach accurate conclusions.

Beliefs, traditions and concepts of our forefathers should be changed if they are found unsuitable in the context of present knowledge. We have to change the concept of religion and spiritualism, arranged marriage system, Homeopathy, Ayurveda, astrology, *tantra mantra*, caste system, exorcism, incantation, etc. if advanced natural science favours change. If we follow the concepts that developed knowledge opposes, it is quite irrational.

"The great Greek physician Hippocrates (460-377 B.C.) has been called the father of modern medicine. He denied the intervention of deities and demons in the development of disease... ." [1] Before Hippocrates it was presumed that all diseases are caused due to supernatural influences. It was Hippocrates who first of all denied supernatural interventions in the development of diseases. He provided revolutionary thought which made him a pioneer of development of the modern medical science.

Not only Hippocrates but many other intellectuals also made successful efforts in the development of therapeutic knowledge. The present knowledge is the cumulative result of these continuous efforts. But one thing is true that right thought and right concept could be determined only after verification by the present developed knowledge. If a concept or a thought cannot be verified by experiments, analyses and arguments, it should be discarded.

Samuel Hahnemann of Germany (1755-1843 A.D.) developed a new system of therapeutics—Homeopathy. It entered India during 1810-1839 and now it has become a part of Indian culture. India has the highest number of Homeopaths in the world. The Homeopathy is also prevalent in some other countries.

In India, Homeopathy is patronized by public as well as by the Government. Indian Government also manages Homeopathy colleges where Homeopathy degrees are awarded. It is a five-year course. Day by day, Homeopathy is becoming popular in India. Physicians of modern medical science also support Homeopathy. They all say, where modern medical science fails, Homeopathy works and it can cure all complicated diseases.

"Homeopathy reached its peak of popularity in the early nineteenth century. Today, there is a resurgence of the popularity of this old medical practice. There are about 3000 recognized practitioners in the US who practice Homeopathy. In the US there are at least five schools and training centers for Homeopathy, 20 Homeopathic pharmacies and four major Homeopathic organizations.

In France, 16 per cent of the population uses Homeopathic drug products on a regular basis. In England, 45 per cent of conventional physicians refer patients to Homeopathic practitioners. In Russia, at least 20 per cent of the medical care is Homeopathic. Homeopathy has a strong following in Belgium, Germany, Netherlands, Italy and South America. Homeopathy traditionally has had a strong following in poorer countries. For example, India has 100,000 prescribers of Homeopathic medicine."[2]

This indicates that Homeopathy is becoming popular throughout the world. But the rules of Homeopathy and the concepts of modern medical science are contradictory to each other. Either modern medical science is correct or Homeopathy is correct. Either modern medical science should be banned or Homeopathy should be discarded. If we are saying that both are correct this indicates our inefficiency and incapability to reach a definite conclusion. If Homeopathy is wrong and it is popular among common men then we, the persons having scientific knowledge, are committing a crime against humanity and science.

My work explaining the fallacies of Homeopathy will help all to reach a definite conclusion.

Rich and resourceful people first take modern medical therapy. In incurable and chronic diseases, they take Homeopathic medicine just for change. They never prefer Homeopathy as a first line treatment. Homeopathy always remains the second alternative method for the rich and educated people. Such illogical use establishes Homeopathy unnecessarily. Poor and uneducated people always prefer Homeopathy because it is cheaper, and then they suffer most. Patients of tuberculosis, malaria, typhoid, etc. die in these families because they were taking Homeopathic medicines for these ailments. There are many glaucomatous blinds in these families because they avoid going for eye surgery and prefer taking Homeopathic drugs. Tuberculosis, leprosy, malaria are increasing day by day because people do not take full course of modern allopathic drugs but shift towards Homeopathy. So drugs are going to be resistant. Homeopathy is a hobby or fashion for richer and resourceful persons but this is a death knell for the poor and uneducated people. Who will be responsible for this? Is scientific community ready to take responsibility for such an offence?

The aim of my work is to find the truth and to protect the poor and uneducated people from dangerous consequences of Homeopathy because people ignore the advantageous medical science. The book intends to remove illogical and wrong concepts from the minds of the people and help in the evolution of logical and scientific knowledge.

In this work I have analysed the principles of Homeopathy, given by Hahnemann. The analysis has been done in the context of present knowledge of medical science.

If Homeopathy is accurate and efficacious then costly modern Allopathy should be replaced by Homeopathy. India is a poor country, then why have we accepted the costly Allopathy?

If Homeopathy is wrong, and treatment of diseases is not possible by Homeopathy, then it should be banned as it is of no use to expend money and time on Homeopathy.

Dinesh Kumar Jain

CONTENTS

BASICS OF HOMEOPATHY

These are the basic principles of Homeopathy. Homeopathy is based on the following conclusions, which are divided into 55 parts.

Hahnemann deduced these conclusions on the basis of his knowledge and his observations:

1. There are two important principles of Homeopathy. The first is "like cures like" which means treatment of disease by the use of a small amount of drug in healthy persons to produce symptoms similar to those of the disease being treated.
2. The second important principle of Homeopathy is dilution and trituration potentiate *the potency of a drug.*
3. Hahnemann criticized Allopathy. In Allopathy, there were a few treatments which were dangerous to human lives. In Allopathy, favourite remedies were blood-letting, emetics and purgatives.
4. According to Homeopathy, knowledge regarding aetiology, pathology and nature of disease is not important.
5. Name and diagnosis of disease are not necessary. Nomenclature of disease is not desired by this system. Knowledge of symptoms is sufficient.
6. Removal of symptoms means total cure. No symptom indicates no disease. Homeopathy says that without symptoms, existence of disease in the body is not possible.
7. Bacteria or other microbial agents, and any other external factors are not responsible for development of disease. According to Homeopathy, dirty food and dirty water cannot be held responsible for any disease.

8. Hahnemann rejected the examination of blood, urine and other investigations for diagnosis and treatment of diseases.
9. Medicines can show nothing curative besides their tendency to produce morbid symptoms in healthy persons and to remove them in diseased persons.
10. Two dissimilar diseases cannot remove or cure each other. Stronger disease only suspends dissimilar weaker disease.
11. Causes of all chronic diseases are only three – **syphilis**, **sycosis** and **psora**.
12. If symptoms of disease are changed then drug should be changed.
13. Hahnemann said, "It is only Homeopathy which can cure disease." Those who believe that there are other therapeutic methods also, do not know Homeopathy.
14. All the curative power of medicines lies in the power of changing the state of man's health, and it is revealed by the observation of the latter. Hahnemann recommended drug of 30th potency for such studies.
15. Artificial disease produced by drugs should be more powerful than natural disease only then can it displace pathological symptoms of disease.
16. *Mercuric chloride* is effective in very dilute concentration and its toxic effect is similar as symptomatology of **syphilis**. It is according to the rules of Homeopathy.
17. Hahnemann observed the effect of *opium* on human beings and saw two types of effects, direct and indirect Both were opposite to each other. He said that firstdirect action was initial aggravation of symptoms. Similar effect was also seenwhen sulphur was given to treat skin diseases.
18. About the year 1500 ... Melampus, a most celebrated physician ... is said to have cured the daughters of Proteus who were affected by wandering **mania**, they were cured chiefly by means of *veratrum album*... . As the plant could also cause **mania**, the story was of twofold interest to Hahnemann.
19. Hahnemann recommended *belladonna* for treatment of **scarlet fever** in an infinitesimal dose because it produces fever. In 1838, the Persian governmentordered doctors to use belladonna in small doses against the epidemics of **scarlet fever** because it was effective. It supported Hahnemann's rule – "like cures like".

20. Clinical experience proved that the medicinal virtues were undoubtedly increased by the process of attenuation, trituration and succussion. By dilution and trituration, effects of *mercury* and *arsenic* are increased. By grinding, insoluble substances become soluble and give colours; that also supports the view that dilution increases power.

21. Allopathic treatment was unscientific, wrong and responsible for more harm than cure. Hahnemann opposed Allopathy and established Homeopathy. One prescription of Hahnemann which made him very popular was treatment of **cholera**. Allopathy was not able to cure the patients of **cholera** but Homeopathy did it.

22. According to Homeopathy, *causes of diseases are actually inside the body*, not outside. Bacteria, viruses, protozoa, mosquitoes, dirty water, unhygienic food and pollution are not responsible for any disease. The basic cause of all diseases is **psora** and that is developed due to wrong thought. Sinful thought and sinful acts are responsible for all chronic diseases. If a person has pure thought, he cannot suffer from any disease. Disease first starts in mind or in psyche or in desire, then it spreads in the body.

23. Jealousy, lack of love, disturbed peace, selfishness, unfairness, unjustified attitude for others are the causative factors in the development of **psora**. **Psora** is the basis of all diseases. Homeopathy divides all diseases into two groups: (1) New, (2) Old. If new diseases are treated wrongly, they convert into old or chronic diseases.

24. Homeopathy opposes external application of lotion or ointment in skin diseases. According to this pathy, skin diseases are not isolated problems, these are actually external manifestations of internal diseases. Local, surgical and other treatments for skin disease are also not indicated in this therapy.

25. **Warts** are cured by internal application of Homeopathic drugs. Localized extirpation of *carcinomatous* growth should not be done because that develops other internal diseases.

26. Rapid increase of psychiatric symptoms is related to improvement in corporal symptoms. Hahnemann prescribed *aconite, belladonna*, *hyoscyamus*, *mercury* in highly potentized minute Homeopathic doses.

27. According to Homeopathy, dilution and trituration increase the potency of a drug. The material part of the medicine is lessened

with each degree of dynamization 50,000 times and yet incredibly increased in power. *The thirtieth thus progressively prepared* would give a fraction almost impossible to be expressedin number but highly potent in power.

28. Homeopathy opposes treatment of fever. **Tuberculosis** and similar diseases are developed when fever is treated. This pathy says that only presence of symptoms indicates the disease. If investigations indicate but there are no symptoms, Homeopathy would not accept the disease. During treatment, first, mind gets cured, only then the body is cured. Homeopaths criticized injections and vaccinations. They say these procedures are very dangerous.
29. If two dissimilar diseases meeting together in the human being are of equal strength or if the older one is stronger, the new disease will be repelled by the old one from the body and not allowed to affect it or strong disease suppresses another weak disease. When stronger disease is cured, weaker disease reappears.
30. In **tuberculosis**, killing of mycobacteria will kill the patient. If we could succeed, today, in putting a fluid into the anatomy it would destroy the bacteria and that consumptive would die soon.
31. Kent said that persons suffering from **diabetes**, **tuberculosis** and **Bright's disease** cannot suffer from dissimilar mild infections like **dysentry**.
32. In Homeopathy, "to know effectiveness of a drug, it should not be given to the patients", because in patients, symptoms produced by drug and symptoms produced by disease will be mixed and then it will be difficult to separate. To know therapeutic effectiveness, drug should be given to healthy persons. In severe acute and chronic diseases which constitute by far the greater portion of all human ailments, crude nature is powerless. In these neither the vital force with its self-aiding faculty nor Allopathy in imitation of it can affect a lysis.
33. Kent concluded that one chronic disease (**syphilis**) suppressed another chronic disease (**Bright's disease**) and when **syphilis** was cured, **Bright's disease** again appeared. Then Kent said "dissimilar are unable to cure, they can only suppress".
34. Homeopathy condemns the principle of the removal of external manifestations of disease by an external means whatsoever.
35. No organ can make the body sick. Man is prior to his organs. Parts of the body can be removed and yet man will exist.

36. How did Hahnemann reach the conclusion that it is not from external things that man becomes sick, not from bacteria, nor environment but from causes in himself. He said intravenous administration of fluid is dangerous to body and bacteria have not been sent on earth to destroy man. Bacteria are perfectlyharmless in every respect.

37. Hahnemann criticized derivation, imitation and counter imitation by saying "it is unhelpful, injurious and indirect mode of treatment". He also opposed large doses which were being used by old allopaths.

38. It is only the slighter and acute disease that tend to terminate quietly in resolution or in death. All chronic diseases of mankind cannot be cured spontaneously. These diseases increase evermore with the years. They never subside on their own but keep increasing and aggravating even till death. There are three chronic diseases: (1) **Syphilis**, (2) **Sycosis**, and (3) **Psora**.

39. **Syphilis** alone has been to some extent known as such a chronic miasmatic disease which when uncured ceases only with the termination of life.

40. Hahnemann writes regarding treatment of **syphilis** that it needs only one little dose of the best *mercurial* remedy in order to cure thoroughly and forever the whole**syphilis** with its **chancre** within 14 days. He also used *arsenic* in treatment of **syphilis** in a single dose.

41. **Sycosis**, the condylomatous disease is ineradicable by the vital force without proper medicinal treatment. **Sycosis** is revealed by cauliflower-like growth. When discharge of **gonorrhoea** is suppressed by allopathic injection, **sycosis** is established in the body.

42. Hahnemann included all venereal diseases into two groups. One where lesion is ulcerative or papular, labelled as **syphilitic** miasm and second, where lesion is like external growth or discharge from the urethra, labelled as **sycosis**. Both were called as two venereal diseases which were treated with the *mercury, thuja* and *nitric acid* by Hahnemann.

43. It had been thought previously that **syphilis** always follows on the destruction of **chancre** by local applications and allopathic drugs modify acute diseases into chronic diseases which become very troublesome to people.

44. Allopathic drugs suppress symptoms to redirect them internally and create various systemic disturbances. By suppression of **psora**, **syphilis** and **sycosis** after administration of allopathic injections, many types of disease symptoms are produced.
45. **Figwart disease** is the result of suppression of **gonorrhoea** by allopathic treatment. Suppression of symptoms increases severity of disease. Kent concluded that allopathic drugs suppress **gonorrhoea** in males and after marriage this suppressed **gonorrhoea** is transmitted to females and causes manysymptoms.
46. Suppressed manifestations must come back and they will come back under appropriate treatment.
47. **Psora** is that most ancient, most universal and most destructive disease which has become the mother of various acute and chronic, non-venereal diseases. The origin of **psora** is related to spiritualism. It is to a spiritual sickness. Wrong thoughts and wrong desires give origin to **psora** and it makes the person susceptible to all diseases.
48. God warned that he should be followed otherwise men will suffer from **tuberculosis** and fever. During evolution, **psora** was in the form of St. Anthony's fire and during the middle ages it reassumed the form of leprosy.
49. After the destruction of external skin eruption, **psora** plays the sad role of causing innumerable secondary symptoms. When skin eruptions subside, severe manifestations are the result. **Psora** spreads from one person to another person. When internal development of **psora** has been completed, vital force develops skin eruption as a substitute for the internal **psora** and keeps the **psora** in confined and stable position.
50. Slumbering and bound **psora** break out due to improper treatment by allopathic physician, through some unlucky physical or psychical occurrence, through a violent fright, continual vexations, deeply affecting grief, catching a severe cold or through a cold temperature, etc. Suppression of itch is mainly responsible for awakening of internal **psora** which gives many chronic **symptomatology** and diseases.
51. Hahnemann presented a list of 97 examples of different clinical manifestations and proved them by simple observation of appearance and disappearance of lesionsthat all clinical problems were due to suppression of itch. There are 15 examples in the list where suppression of **tinea** complex results in secondary diseases.

52. Time interval is different in different cases after the suppression of itch and development of secondary diseases. **Epilepsy** and fever also developed due to suppression of itch. Reappearance of itch and eruption is a must for cure.

53. Hahnemann himself quoted examples where without applying external allopathic treatment, eruptions were suppressed and created secondary clinical symptoms.

54. New medicine and new dose of the same medicine would interrupt the work of improvement and cause new ailments which often cannot be repaired for a long time. If somebody does this, he is unworthy of a Homeopathic physician. In exceptional cases, repetition of dose is allowed but in different potency.Homeopathic drugs are effective also by respiratory route. When the treatment of infant is concerned, Hahnemann advised drug administration to the nursing mother.

55. Hahnemann accepted failure of Homeopathic treatment. He said that he was not able to cure all chronic patients. He mentioned many factors which make patients incurable and augment their diseases.

HOMEOPATHIC CONCEPTS

1

There are two important principles of Homeopathy. The first is "like cures like" which means treatment of disease by the use of a small amount of drug that in healthy persons to produce symptoms similar to those of the disease being treated.

ARGUMENT

"There are two important principles of Homeopathy."[3] The first is "like cures like" which means symptoms of disease can be reproduced in a healthy body by a drug then this drug is effective in that disease. Similar symptoms in the remedy remove similar symptoms in the disease. The universal law of nature is that every disease is destroyed and cured through the similar artificial disease which the appropriate remedy has the tendency to excite. Among two similar diseases only one disease can exist in the body at any one time.

The second important principle of Homeopathy is "dilution potentiates the potency". According to Hahnemann, "effect of drugs is potentiated by dilution even to the extent that an effective dose may not contain a single molecule of drug. Hahnemann recommended 30th potency dilution in which"[4] one molecule of drug would be in a volume of a sphere of literally astronomical circumference.

Both these principles of Homeopathy were analysed and it was found that the conclusion drawn by Hahnemann was wrong. "Hahnemann's first principle was a generalization based on the fact that a large dose of *cinchona bark* induced in him a **malarial** paroxysm. The reason for this occurrence being that he had previously suffered from **malaria** and the gastric irritation excited the paroxysm."[5]

Hahnemann could not understand this fact that he had suffered from **malaria** and gastric irritation by *cinchona bark* which was responsible for his recurrence of paroxysm.

The *cinchona bark* contains *quinine* alkaloid. This alkaloid has antimalarial action. "In **malarial** fever, *quinine* has a direct action on the organism causing the disease and suppresses the elevated body temperature. *Quinine* may exercise a true antipyretic action. The effect of *quinine* on normal body temperature is negligible."[6]

"*Quinine* has an analgesic and antipyretic action and a definite lowering of body temperature occurs in fever from any cause. For this reason *quinine* has been used in many symptomatic remedies."[7]

"Rigors or chills, are common at the onset of various febrile disorders and may occur at regular or irregular intervals. The cardinal feature of rigor is shivering. Chills and rigors may be produced and perpetuated by intermittent administration of an effective antipyretic agent. This may cause a sharp depression of a raised temperature in a febrile state, which precipitates involuntary muscular contraction."[8]

"Initially rigors also occur in acute gastrointestinal disorder."[9]

Relapses of **malaria** occur when "Malarial parasites (Exo erythrocytic) persisting in the liver reinvade the blood stream and patients should be followed for one month to detect recrudescence of the infection."[10] Form of malarial parasites persisting in the liver is not destroyed by *quinine* present in *cinchona bark.*

It was observed that "**Malaria** may remain latent for many years. Reappearance is brought about by cold, general depression of health or through some intercurrent malady."[11]

The main constituent of *cinchona bark* is *quinine.* "Oral administration of *quinine* often results in nausea, vomiting and epigastric pain."[12]

By these observations from medical science we can conclude as follows:

1. *Quinine* is the main component of *cinchona bark* which is effective against **malarial** fever. The effect of *quinine* on normal body temperature is negligible.
2. Hahnemann had suffered from **malaria**. Just after this, he took *cinchona bark* and got **malarial** paroxysm. The cause of this incidence can be explained as:

(*a*) Within one month of malarial attack, chances of **malaria** relapse is very high. Relapse may occur by acute gastrointestinal problem or any intercurrent malady. Hahnemann had taken *cinchona* after symptomatic cure of **malaria**. Gastrointestinal problem created by *cinchona* could be responsible for recurrence of **malarial** paroxysm.

Normal body temperature is not altered and **malarial** paroxysm does not occur in normal healthy person after taking *cinchona.*

(*b*) Second explanation can also be given for recurrence of **malarial** paroxysm. At the time of Hahnemann, the actual cause of **malaria** was not known. "Ronald Ross discovered the transmission of **malaria** by Anopheline mosquitoes in 1897 and also discovered malarial parasites. Plasmodium responsible for malarial attack and diagnosis of malaria depends on demonstration of the parasite in the blood."[13] The paroxysm of fever with chill, which Hahnemann suffered after taking *cinchona,* might not be malaria, because at that time cause of malaria was not known. So confirmation of **malaria** was not possible by demonstration of malarial parasite in blood. There are so many causes of fever with chills. It might be possible that Hahnemann had suffered from other disease having symptoms of fever with chill. It was just coincidence that at that time he took *cinchona* and he wrongly concluded that this paroxysm was of **malaria** and due to *cinchona.*

If principle of Homeopathy is true then *quinine* should produce rigors in healthy body. But study says that *quinine* does not produce rigors. If Hahnemann is true then *quinine* should produce rigours in healthy body because *quinine* is effective in **malaria** which is characterized by rigors with fever.

I will write again that in medical science conclusion cannot be drawn by single observation or observation in few persons. Those doctors who believe in single observation or observation in a few persons and draw conclusion on this basis only, don't know anything regarding medical science.

During single observation or observation in single or few persons, there are various factors which may influence observation and give wrong conclusion.

Hahnemann and his followers did this mistake. In therapeutics, controlled experiments in hundred and thousands of patients are done to draw the right conclusion.

2

The second important principle of Homeopathy is dilution and trituration potentiate the potency of a drug.

ARGUMENT

Second important principle of Homeopathy is "dilution **potentiates** the potency". Hahnemann derived this principle by the following observation and experiment.

Hahnemann found that "**trituration** of *mercury* increased its pharmacological effect".[14] He observed that potency of *mercury* was increased after dilution and **trituration**. Later on this conclusion was analysed and it was found that increased potency of *mercury* was not due to dilute and triturated *mercury*.

"This increased effect was due to oxidation of *mercury*, first to *mercurous* and later to *mercuric oxide*."[15]

The **potentiated** effect, that Hahnemann observed was due to mercuric oxide.

This second important principle of Homeopathy again was due to wrong generalization of wrong observation.

Today it is also known that "elemental *mercury* cannot react with biologically important molecules. When ingested or taken orally, it occurs as large globular particles in the G.I.T. and is absorbed very poorly. The soluble inorganic *mercuric salts* gain access to the circulation when taken orally".[16] It has also been found that "*mercury* is easily converted into the form of a dull grey powder when triturated with sugar, chalk or lard. The process is known as deadening. Grey powder contains 33 per cent of *mercury* and a portion of the *mercury* is converted into *mercuric oxide* which produces a poisonous action on the system".[17]

"Cases are recorded where individuals have swallowed a pound or two of the liquid metal (perfectly pure) without any harmful effect."[18]

"The *salts of mercury* and *silver* dissolved in water have been used as antiseptic solutions for many years. Today these substances have to a large extent been replaced by less toxic organic chemicals. Solutions of *mercuric chloride* are useful in disinfecting materials. Aqueous solutions of 1:100 to 1:10000 dilutions are generally employed."[19]

Now it is very clear that *mercury* in pure form is an inert substance when given orally but mercuric compounds obtained after **trituration** of *mercury* is highly potent and effective in more dilutions.

Now it can be said that it was not dilution and **trituration** which increased potency of *mercury*; it was actually conversion of mercury into *mercuric oxide* which was responsible for increased potency. Now we are taking another parameter. If dilution increases potency then dilute drugs should have stronger action than concentrated drugs. Observations do not prove this statement.

Observations in patients prove that concentrated drugs have stronger and more potent action than dilute drugs. Few examples are being given. *Methylmercury* in blood produces various manifestations. Blood concentration of 0.1-0.5 ng/ml produces no ataxia, no visual defect, no hearing defect and no death. Blood concentration of 1-2 ng/ml of *methyl mercury* causes ataxia in 47 per cent persons, visual defect in 53 per cent cases, hearing defect in 5 per cent cases and no death; while blood concentration of 4-5 ng/ml produces ataxia in 100 per cent cases, visual defect in 83 per cent cases, hearing defect in 66 per cent cases and death in 28 per cent cases."[20]

Behavior and physiological effects of *ethanol* in human associated with increasing blood *ethanol* concentration also proves that Hahnemann's principle of dilution is wrong. When *ethanol* concentration of blood is increased, toxic effects are also increased while Hahnemann said dilution increases potency of a drug:

"Blood ethanol concentration	*Nature of effect*
<50 mg/dl	Increased sociability, euphoria
50-100 mg/dl	Disturbance in gait, lack of concentration, increased reaction time
100-150 mg/dl	Ataxia, impaired motor and mental skills. Slurred speech
200 mg/dl	No response to sensory stimuli
250 mg/dl	Coma
500 mg/dl	Death"[21]

"Plasma concentration of *Lithium* in **mania** should range from 0.9 to 1.4 mEq/L. Concentration higher than 1.5 mEq/L is associated with an increased incidence of side effects, while those about 2 mEq/L may result in serious toxicity."[22]

Now it is clear that dilution does not increase potency.

"From 1829 onward Hahnemann recommended the administration of all drugs at the thirtieth potency which corresponds to a concentration of 1 part in 10^{60} parts. This works out at a content of 1 molecule of drug in a sphere with a circumference equal to the orbit of Neptune."[23]

The distance between Neptune and sun is 4496.6×10^6 kilometer. This is the radius of sphere produced by Neptune around the sun. The volume of this sphere will be $4/3\ \pi r^3$. It will be equal to

$$\frac{4}{3}\times\frac{22}{7}\times(4496.6\times10^6)^3$$

$$= \frac{4}{3}\times\frac{22}{7}\times\frac{4496.6}{1}\times\frac{4496.6}{1}\times\frac{4496.6}{1}\times10^{18}$$

$$= 364\times10^{27} \text{ cubic km. approximately}$$

We can conclude that a container of 70,000 lac kilometer length, 70,000 lac kilometer width and 70,000 lac kilometer height, which is filled with Homeopathic drug of 30th potency will contain only 1 molecule of Homeopathic drug.

We can also explain in another way. If we give Homeopathic drug to a patient in that amount which is equal to the water contained in all the rivers and oceans on the earth will not contain any molecule of drug. We can also say that the amount of Homeopathic drug given to the patients contains no drug at all.

3

Hahnemann criticized Allopathy. In Allopathy, there were a few treatments which were dangerous to human lives. In Allopathy the favourite remedies were bloodletting, emetics and purgatives.

ARGUMENT

Hahnemann said in 1842 that Allopathy was wrong. He criticized Allopathy. Now here is a question what was that Allopathy, which was criticized by Hahnemann. Was it modern medical science or some other method of therapeutics? Followers of Hahnemann today criticize modern medical science on the basis of Homeopathic principles. Are they correct or are they giving wrong messages to the public? These are very important questions which everybody should know.

The word Homeopathy indicates – *homeo* = similar, *pathos* = suffering. The symptoms produced by drugs are similar to the symptoms of disease. That's why this system of therapeutics was known as Homeopathy. The word Allopathy consists of allo and pathos. *Allo* means different and *pathos* means suffering. Here the symptoms produced by the drugs are different than that of the disease. Therefore, this system of medicine was known as Allopathy.

What was Allopathy in the year 1800? "In Allopathy, favourite remedies were bloodletting, emetics and purgatives and these were used until the dominant symptoms of the disease were suppressed. **Malaria** and **dysentery** were treated by purging with *calomel* until collapse was produced. In large proportion of cases the suppression of the symptoms by collapse was followed shortly by death."[24]

In the year 1827, bloodletting was done by leech in Allopathy. Thirty two million leeches were used in France. This system of Allopathy was not based on an adequate knowledge of physiology and pathology. It was responsible for the death of many patients instead of curing.

"Bloodletting is also a part of Ayurveda. Leeches are used in Ayurveda for this purpose. Even today leeches are being used in Ayurveda hospitals in India for bloodletting. It has been said that many skin diseases are cured by this procedure and this application is a part of Ayurveda."[25]

Hahnemann criticized Allopathy because leeches were being used. Today, leeches are being used in Ayurveda hospitals in India. Actually Ayurveda was also a part of old Allopathy which was criticized by Hahnemann. I am sorry to say that today people are accepting both Ayurveda and Homeopathy without understanding that both are also opposite to each other.

Hahnemann rightly criticized Allopathy. Hahnemann writes "Allopathy knows no treatment except to draw from diseases the injurious materials which are assumed to be their cause. The blood of the patient is made to flow mercilessly by bleedings, leeches cuppings to diminish an assumed plethora (excess of blood) ... while the loss of blood ... destroys life. Allopathy taps off the life's blood and exerts itself either to clear away the imaginary disease matter or to conduct it elsewhere (by emetics, purgatives, diuretics, drawing plasters). This renders incurable, if not fatal, the majority of diseases. Patient's sufferings are thereby increased and by such and other painful appliances the forces and nutritious juices indispensable to the curative process are abstracted from the organism."[26]

Hahnemann has also written:

"Allopathy has shortened the *lives of ten times* as many human beings as the most destructive wars and rendered many millions of patients more diseased and wretched than they were originally."[27]

Whatever Samuel Hahnemann said in 1840 about Allopathy was right but what his followers are saying today is absolutely wrong. Today, followers of Homeopathy criticize modern medical science. They use the word Allopathy for it. This is wrong. Modern medical science is not related with old Allopathy. The use of term 'Allopathy' for modern medical science is wrong. But it is a common practice to use the term Allopathy for modern medical science. In fact principles of old Allopathy are different from modern medical science. Basis of old Allopathy were neither logical nor correct.

Modern medical science is based on logical, controlled, accurate experimentation with full knowledge of pathogenesis of disease, pharmacokinetic and pharmacodynamic study of drugs. In his full work and everywhere Hahnemann criticized Allopathy. This criticism is not related with modern medical science in any way.

Hahnemann writes:

"Use of *calomel, corrosive sublimate, mercurial ointment, nitrate of silver, iodine ointment, opium, valerian, cinchona bark* and *quinine, fox glove, prussic acid, sulphur* and *sulphuric acid,* venesections, shedding streams of blood, leeches is dangerous to human body."[28] These drugs and treatment were used by old Allopathy. Now in present medical science these treatments are not used systemically. Locally some compounds are used. Criticism of these treatments by Hahnemann is correct. But present medical science or present Allopathy does not permit use of these treatments. Only *quinine* and *iodine* are used systemically in *malaria* and *hypothyroidism* respectively. Modern medical science uses *iodine* or *quinine* only after extensive study of 5 to 10 years on these compounds.

Hahnemann "Said about Allopathy"[29] that this pathy is useless, cannot treat the disease, and creates various problems in the body and makes diseases incurable. He also says, innumerable abnormal conditions are produced by Allopathy which cannot be treated.

I am again and again saying that it was the criticism of old Allopathic mode of treatment. This criticism is right but not related with modern medical science which is also wrongly named Allopathy today.

4

According to Homeopathy, knowledge regarding aetiology, pathology and nature of disease is not important.

ARGUMENT

What Hahnemann emphasized in his first direction is:

"The physician's high and only mission is to restore the sick to health, to cure. His mission is not however to construct so-called systems ... and hypothesis concerning the internal essential nature of the vital process and the mode in which diseases originate in the invisible interior of the organism, nor is it to attempt to give countless explanations regarding the phenomenon in diseases and their proximate cause."[30]

According to Homeopathy, knowledge and research regarding aetiology, pathology and nature of disease is not important. It is a wastage of time and talent. Due to this, Homeopathy blocked development of medical knowledge. Side by side, it also indicates that in Homeopathy, knowledge regarding aetiology, pathology and prognosis is not required. In this way questions against Homeopathy cannot be raised on the basis of knowledge of developed medical science. It is ridiculous.

Aetiology of disease is important to determine method of treatment. Pathogenesis is important to know accurate mechanism of symptomatology. The diagnosis of disease is also important to treat it accurately. Investigations are helpful in diagnosis. The discovery of new drugs also depends on detailed knowledge of diseases. Homeopathy opposes detailed study of diseases. However, without knowledge of aetiology, prevention of disease cannot be possible. Today, we know that preventive aspect of disease is more important than curative aspect. Many diseases like **AIDS**, **rabies**, have no cure. Only prevention of these diseases are possible and that can be done only on the basis of knowledge regarding aetiology and pathogenesis. All communicable diseases can be prevented in this manner. Prevention is thus advised only by modern medical science and not by Homeopathy.

5

> Name and diagnosis of disease are not necessary. Nomenclature of disease is not desired by this system. Knowledge of symptoms is sufficient.

ARGUMENT

Homeopathy says, "Name and diagnosis of disease is not necessary. Nomenclature of disease is not desired by this system. Knowledge of symptoms is sufficient in this therapy."[31] This indicates that diseases having common symptoms will be treated by a single drug. In Homeopathy aetiology is not important for treatment purpose. Causative agent may be bacterial, fungal, hormonal or carcinomatous but treatment in Homeopathy will remain same. It is again an illogical concept.

I am writing one example. **Neurocysticercosis**, **tuberculoma** of brain and **neoplasm** in the brain, all these three diseases may have similar symptoms but the treatment part is quite different.

Other important examples are headache, chest pain, dyspnoea, and pain in abdomen. Each symptom has many causes which represent different diseases. Different diseases require different treatment. If all patients with similar symptoms are treated by single drug, cure is never possible.

6

Removal of symptoms means total cure. No symptom indicates no disease. Without symptoms existence of disease in the body is not possible, says Homeopathy.

ARGUMENT

The other basic concept of Homeopathy is:

"It is not conceivable, nor can it be proved by any experience in the world, that after removal of all the symptoms of the disease ... there should or could remain anything else besides health or that the morbid alteration in the interior could remain uneradicated."[32] In this paragraph it is said, if symptoms of a disease are removed, disease is cured. Without symptoms disease cannot exist in the body. But today we know by the help of developed medical science that there are many diseases which have no symptoms at their early stage. Pathogenesis starts during the early stage. Healthy state of body is changed but there is no symptom. As diseases advance, symptoms appear. Many diseases are episodic in nature. Between the episodes, patient has no symptoms at all, although diseases persist in the body. **Hypertension** (a cardiovascular disease) may not produce any symptom even at an advanced stage, that's why it has been called a silent killer.

Similarly a form of **myocardial infarction** called silent **myocardial infarction** is asymptomatic, although it may prove fatal. **Carcinoma, diabetes, degenerative neurological disease** do not have any symptoms during their early stage. Diseases like **asthma**, **epilepsy**, **angina** and **peptic ulcer** are episodic in nature, with symptom-free periods between attacks.

Now it can be said that without symptoms, existence of disease in the body is possible. It is against the basic concept of Homeopathy.

7

Bacteria or other microbial agents, and any other external factor are not responsible for development of disease. According to Homeopathy, dirty food and dirty water cannot be held responsible for any disease.

ARGUMENT

One of the most important concept of Homeopathy is regarding causative factors of disease. According to Homeopathy, "Bacteria are not causative factors in disease."[33]

Kent says:

"The bacteria are results of disease ... microscopical little fellows do not cause the disease, but that they come after, that they are scavengers accompanying the disease and that they are perfectly harmless in every respect. They are the outcome of the disease and present wherever the disease is ... ."[34]

Kent further states:

"It is not from external things that man becomes sick neither from bacteria nor environment but from causes in himself. If the Homeopath does not see this, he cannot have a true perception of the disease. Disorder in the vital economy is the primary state of affairs and this disorder manifests itself by signs and symptoms."[35]

Now it is clear that according to Homeopathy, bacteria and other external agents like viruses, fungi, parasites, worms and pollutants are not causative factors. Today, it has been absolutely proved that "bacteria, viruses, fungi worms, and pollutants cause various diseases."[36] In India 75 to 85 per cent of diseases are caused by these agents.**Typhoid**, **cholera**, **bacillary dysentery**, **pneumonia**, **respiratory tract infections**, **urinary tract infections**, **meningitis**, **tuberculosis**, **leprosy**, are common bacterial diseases about which even a lay person knows that these are caused by bacteria. These diseases can only be treated by those drugs which kill responsible pathogens.

These are few examples of bacteria responsible for diseases: "Mycobacterium tuberculosis causes **tuberculosis**, mycobacterium leprae causes **leprosy**, legionella causes **legionnaires disease**, calymmatobacterium granulomatis causes **granuloma inguinale**, haemophilus ducrezi causes **chancroid**, salmonella bacteria causes **typhoid fever**, clostridium tetani causes **tetanus**. Similarly other organisms are spirochetes, fungus, virus, etc. which also produce diseases. Trepanoma pallidum produces **syphilis**, trepanoma pertenue produces **yaws,** leptospira produces **Weil's disease**, chlamydia trachomatis produces **trachoma**. Various viruses like HIV virus produces **AIDS** disease, influenza virus produces **influenza**. In the absence of these organisms respective diseases cannot be produced."[37]

Antibiotics are drugs used for killing these bacteria. Antibiotics kill bacteria that's why they are used in diseases caused by bacteria. *Chloramphenicol, Amoxycillm, Cotrimoxazole* are used in **typhoid** because these drugs kill salmonella bacteria. "Approximately 30 per cent of all hospitalized patients receive one or more courses of therapy with antibiotics and millions of potentially fatal infections have been cured.'[38]

"When an antimicrobial agent is indicated, the goal is to choose a drug that is selective for the infecting micro-organism.'[39]

"A large percentage of antibiotics administered in the United States are given to prevent infections rather than to treat established disease."[40]

Now it is clear that antibiotics kill bacteria and cure diseases. Antibiotics also prevent development of disease in the body that's why they are also used for prophylaxis. It has also been proved by animal experiments that bacteria, viruses, fungi, spirochaetes are responsible for various diseases. These are definite causative factors in disease production. Homeopathy says bacteria and virus like organisms are not causative factors in disease. Now we can say, this Homeopathic concept is wrong. Pathology is the subject where pathogenesis is taught. Pathogenesis means how diseases are developed by bacteria, virus and other causative factors.

"Pathology is the study of disease by scientific methods. Disease may be defined as an abnormal variation in the structure or function of any part of the body. In other words, diseases have causes."[41] "Causative factors in disease may be of a genetic nature or acquired. Acquired disease is due to effects of some environmental factors. Parasitic micro-organisms include bacteria, protozoa, lower fungi and viruses. The disease-producing capacity of micro-organisms depend on their ability to invade and multiply within the host. Bacteria bring about harmful effects mainly by the production of chemical compounds termed as toxins."[42] It is also true that "Infective disease was the major cause of death throughout the world, and the elimination or reduction in the incidence of most of the important infections largely accounts for the greatly increased lifespan in technologically advanced communities."[43]

"Infective diseases are still of considerable importance. It remains the major cause of death in many tropical and subtropical countries where in addition to bacterial and viral infection protozoal and metazoal parasites account for a great deal of illness."[44]

If bacteria are not responsible for diseases, then transmission of bacteria from one person to another person cannot produce similar disease but "communicable disease is transmitted via direct transmission like direct contact, droplet infection, contact with soil, inoculation into skin and through placenta and via indirect transmission like vehicle borne, vector borne, air borne, fomite borne and by unclean hands and fingers."[45] This proves that transmission of bacteria from one person to another produces similar disease.

Inoculation of bacteria in animals produces similar disease as produced in human beings also confirms that bacteria causes disease. A person infected with HIV virus will develop **AIDS** and a person not infected with HIV virus will not develop **AIDS** disease also confirms the same thing. If it is confirmed in lab that a particular bacteria is resistant to a drug then this drug will not be effective in disease produced by that bacteria. This also gives same conclusion.

The spread of communicable disease can also be checked by preventing transmission of aetiological agent. Spread of **cholera** can be prevented by purifying contaminated food and water. Spread of **malaria** can be checked by preventing mosquito bite. If **cholera**, **typhoid** and

malaria originate from within the body then these diseases cannot be checked by preventing transmission of bacteria and malarial parasite.

Now, a conclusion can be drawn that bacteria, virus and parasites are definite causative factors in disease. Homeopathy says bacteria, virus and any other external agent are not causative factors in disease. What does this indicate? This indicates that concepts of Homeopathy are not correct.

8

Hahnemann rejected the examination of blood, urine and other investigations for diagnosis and treatment of diseases.

ARGUMENT

Hahnemann says that "Totality of the symptoms is the only indication, the only guide to the selection of a remedy."[46]

"Only on the basis of symptoms drug should be selected. There is no other alternative for drug selection. Hahnemann rejected the examination of blood, urine, and other investigation for diagnosis and treatment of disease."[47]

Here Hahnemann is absolutely wrong. There are various examples which are against this view. Causes of fever are many.

"Bacterial, viral, malarial parasite, rickettsias, chlamydia are infections responsible for fever. Mechanical trauma, neoplasm, hematopoietic disorder, vascular accidents and acute metabolic disorder also cause fever."[48]

Without full investigation it is not possible to diagnose fever and without accurate diagnosis it is not possible to treat fever. Accurate diagnosis is done on the basis of investigations only. If somebody says that on the basis of symptoms only can he diagnose all diseases, he does not know anything regarding medical science.

Similar to fever there are many diseases having common symptoms which cannot be treated without accurate diagnosis and such diagnosis solely depends on various investigations. Hahnemann writes:

"Physician can discover diseases solely of the totality of the symptoms by means of which the disease demands the medicine requisite for its relief, whilst on the other hand every internal cause attributed to it, every occult quality or imaginary material morbific principle is nothing but an idle dream."[49]

According to Homeopathy, there is no need to discover any internal cause of disease and any external bacteria or virus. The study of symptoms is sufficient. For example, if a patient is suffering from abdominal pain, there is no need of investigation like ultrasound or X-ray.

Investigations are not required in Homeopathy. Abdominal pain may be due to pathology in liver or pancreas or stomach or duodenum or uterus or ovary or cardiac or muscular organs. In Homeopathy, it is not required to know which organ is responsible for pain. In Homeopathy, it is also undesirable to know which organ has pathology. Irrespective of organ pathology and irrespective of cause in Homeopathy, treatment of abdominal pain remains constant and in this therapy treatment would be done by that drug which will cause abdominal pain in healthy body.

In a tropical country like India, conditions are quite different as maximum number of diseases are due to micro-organisms. In viral and bacterial diseases immunity plays an important role in recovery. Viral diseases usually resolve spontaneously. This is also true for many bacterial diseases. Many sexually transmitted diseases are also cured spontaneously. When diseases are going to be resolved spontaneously then neither diagnosis nor treatment is important. In these diseases, like Homeopathy, many other systems get unnecessary reputation as curative methods without having any useful therapeutic action. When diseases have to be cured spontaneously then it is not important that diagnosis is not being made and pseudo-treatment is being given. Due to this, Hahnemann got unnecessary reputation and he formulated a wrong concept that the study of symptoms is sufficient and investigations are not required.

9

Medicines can show nothing curative besides their tendency to produce morbid symptoms in healthy persons and to remove them in diseased persons.

ARGUMENT

Homeopathy says: "It is very evident that medicines could never cure diseases if they did not possess the power of altering man's state of health. Their curative power must be owing solely to this power they possess of altering man's state of health."[50] Homeopathy also says that "medicines can show nothing curative besides their tendency to produce morbid symptoms in healthy persons and to remove them in diseased persons."[51]

This indicates that according to Homeopathy, if a drug is not able to produce side effects in a healthy person, it will not be able to cure disease. But Ayurveda says that Ayurvedic drugs do not have any side effects and these drugs have only therapeutic effect. This is a contradiction between Ayurvedic and Homeopathic drugs. But people accept Ayurveda and Homeopathy both without any logical thinking.

According to Homeopathy, there are two different systems of treatment. One is Homeopathy where symptoms produced by drug in healthy body are similar as symptoms of disease. In another system symptoms produced by drug in healthy body are neither similar nor opposite but quite heterogeneous to the symptoms of the disease. This system is known as Allopathic method of therapy.

"Allopathic method of treatment includes Ayurveda and Yunani system."[52] Here again, Homeopathy and Ayurveda have opposite concepts but people accept and favour both Ayurveda and Homeopathy without knowing the basics.

Homeopathy also says—"Nothing can be observed that can constitute them medicine or remedies except that power of causing distinct alteration on the state of health of human body."[53] In 1833, when Hahnemann wrote *Organon of Medicine*, there was nothing except development of morbid symptoms in healthy body by a drug to test its therapeutic capability because at that time there were no biochemical tests, no histopathological study, no culture and sensitivity study, no biopsy, no X-rays, no ultrasound, no M.R.I. In the absence of knowledge, Hahnemann made hypothetical and philosophical concepts which were not based on scientific observations.

Therapeutic potency of a drug cannot be evaluated by morbid alteration in a healthy body.

Hahnemann writes—"Each individual case of disease is most surely, radically, rapidly and permanently annihilated and removed only by a medicine capable of producing in the human system in the most similar and complete manner the totality of its symptoms, which at the same time are stronger than the disease."[54]

Hahnemann writes—"No other mode of employing medicines in diseases that promises to be of service besides the Homeopathic ... a medicine which among all medicines has the power and the tendency to produce an artificial morbid state most similar to that of the case of disease in question."[55]

Today, we have various examples of drugs which do not prove Homeopathic concept. "Antipsychotic drugs like *chlorpromazine, thioridazine* are useful in **Schizophrenia**, but when these drugs are given to healthy individuals, they never produce symptoms of **schizophrenia**. Similarly antidepressant drugs like *imipramine* and *amitryptiline* used in **depression** never produce **depression** in healthy persons. *Antacids* are used in hyperacidity and these drugs never produce hyperacidity in healthy individuals. Various antibiotics like *Ampicillin*, *erythromycins* are used in *respiratory tract infections* but they never develop symptoms of **respiratory infections** in healthy people."[56] Similarly there are various examples which prove that Homeopathic concepts which are given above are wrong. Antileprosy drug cures **leprosy** but never produces **leprosy** in healthy persons. Antitubercular drugs cure **tuberculosis** but these drugs never give symptoms of **tuberculosis** when given to healthy person. Antihypertensive drugs never produce **hypertensive state** when given to a normal healthy body. Drugs used for pain like *brufen* never produce pain in healthy human.

Similarly "Combination of *trimethoprim* and *sulfamethoxazole* is useful in **typhoid** but this combination never produces symptoms of **typhoid** when given to a healthy individual. Another example is *ciprofloxacin* which is used in so many diseases related to urinary tract, prostate, respiratory tract, bone, gastrointestinal tract but never produces symptoms of these diseases."[57]

Hahnemann further writes—"Medicine should be capable of producing in the human body an artificial disease as similar as possible to the disease to be cured which with somewhat increased power."[58]

By the help of above examples, it can be said that drugs useful in a particular disease neither produce symptoms of that disease in healthy individuals nor produces artificial disease, similar to the disease to be cured. In this way we can say that the above given statements of Hahnemann are not correct.

10

Two dissimilar diseases cannot remove or cure each other. Stronger disease only suspends dissimilar weaker disease.

ARGUMENT

Hahnemann writes—"If new dissimilar disease is stronger than the disease under which the patient originally labored being the weaker will be kept back and suspended by the accession of the stronger one, until the later shall have run its course or been cured and then the old one reappears uncured."[59]

I am saying repeatedly that by the help of one, two or few examples in medical science, any conclusion cannot be drawn. It could be by chance.

For example, Hahnemann quoted— "Two children affected with a kind of **epilepsy** remained free from **epileptic attacks** after infection with **ringworm** but as soon as eruption on head was gone, the**epilepsy** returned just as before."[59] Here Hahnemann made a wrong conclusion of suspension of **epilepsy** by **ringworm**. The fact is different. Actually in **epilepsy**, attack occurs intermittently with the gap of days, weeks or months. It is the natural course of the disease. During the middle silent stage of **epilepsy** if **ringworm** appears and subsides then how can the relation between **epilepsy** and **ringworm** be established. To establish such relation is useless.

Hahnemann made some observations of infective diseases. He found that sometimes one disease suspended another disease and sometimes one disease cured another disease. He did not know about the mechanism of immunity and antigen—antibody reaction which plays a main part in suspending and curing one disease by another. The important points of this process are being given here:

(*a*) Following immunization (or by a disease) a disease may occur totally unconnected with the immunizing agent (or disease producing agent). Actually the individual is harbouring the infectious agent and administration of vaccine or exposure to disease shorten the incubation period and produces the disease, in such cases.

(*b*) If many antigens are administered into an animal at the same time, the antibody response to each may be less than that if the antigens are introduced individually.

(*c*) "Recovery is of course the rule in the vast majority of viral infections."[60]

(*d*) Cox virus and smallpox virus have common antigens and give immunity to each other.

(*e*) One or few observations do not give any clue.

(*f*) First we should know the normal course of the disease then only we can study the influence of other factors on disease process.

(*g*) "Many infections (viral) are entirely *symptomless* and immunity to reinfection is acquired without serious disturbance at the time of primary infection although latent infection with virus may continue for months or occasionally even for years."[61]

(*h*) "Persistent virus infections are known to occur in man ... slow virus infections may be defined as virus disease having a long incubation period, in some instance years ... in a few virus disease reinfection or repeated infections are common. This may be due to the existence of numerous serologically distinct strain of virus."[62]

(*i*) "Virus infections occur with disease or asymptomatics. The severity of disease may also be age related. In adults **chicken pox** and **mumps** are often severe with complications which are rare during childhood."[63]

(*j*) "If common exposure of viral infection to several persons occurs, illness may be simultaneous irrespective of the length of the incubation period."[64]

(*k*) Diagnosis of viral disease is only done by isolation or recognition of virus and by the help of specific serological tests.

(*l*) "In the acute phase of virus infections a protein *interferon* can be detected in blood and tissue. *Interferon* is released from cells in response to virus infections and when taken up by other cells make them refractory to virus infection. It is not virus specific in its antiviral effect but inhibits virtually all viruses. It begins to appear in bloodstream only when the acute infection is subsiding."[65]

By the help of the above information we can understand causes of varied incubation period, duration, intensity and prognosis of a disease when patient also suffers with another disease. In favour of his opinion Hahnemann writes—"During an epidemic, in which **smallpox** and **measles** were prevalent at the same time, these diseases avoided or suspended one another."[66] Actually both are viral infections and *interferon* produced by acute viral infection prevented or suspended another viral infection.

"Simultaneous occurrence of **smallpox** and **measles** also occur at the same time as written by Hahnemann",[67] in this case *interferon* is not in sufficient amount which could have suspended second infection.

In another case "**Measles** suspended the **cowpox**."[68] In another example "Even after **measles** had broken out the **cowpox** inoculation took effect but did not run its course until the **measles** had disappeared."[69] In other example "**Mumps** immediately disappear when the **cowpox** inoculation had taken effect and had nearly attained its height, it was not until the complete termination of the **cowpox** ... **mumps** reappeared and ran its regular course of seven days."[70]

Hahnemann also writes—"**Smallpox** cures swelling of testicle and in one observation a large hard swelling of the left testicle consequent on a bruise is cured by **smallpox**."[71] It is normal observation that after trauma, swelling anywhere in body is resolved automatically. Similarly, swelling in testicle after trauma is cured automatically. This cure is not related with **smallpox**. The relation between swelling induced by trauma and **smallpox** infection is incorrect. Other examples mentioned by Hahnemann in favour of his view, are being analyzed in the last portion of this book.

One viral infection may suspend or prevent second subsequent infection due to common antigenic structure or release of *interferon*. Similarity or dissimilarity of symptomatology in these two diseases are not important. Only those infective organisms which produce *interferon* may prevent another viral infection, because *interferon* has antiviral action. Many infective and non-infective diseases having dissimilar symptomatology coexist together in the body, such examples are being given in argument no. 29. Again Hahnemann made a wrong generalization of the few observations.

11

Causes of all chronic diseases are only three—**syphilis**, **sycosis** and **psora**.

ARGUMENT

"Hahnemann says that fundamental causes of all chronic diseases are three—(1) **Syphilis**, (2) **Sycosis** and (3) **Psora**. Hahnemann further says that even after treatment of skin eruption of **syphilis** and **sycosis,** seeds of these diseases remain inside the body and continuously create problems. **Syphilis** reveals its specific internal **dyscrasia** by venereal chancre and **sycosis** by cauliflower-like growth and sometimes also causes skin eruption with itching. Third, **psora** is a more dangerous seed than **syphilis** and **sycosis**. This is the only real fundamental cause and producer of numerous innumerable forms of diseases. According to Hahnemann, nervous debility, **hysteria**, **hypochondriasis, mania**, **melancholia, imbecility, madness, epilepsy, convulsion of all sorts**, **softening of bone**, **scoliosis**, **caries**, **cancer**, **neoplasm**, **gout**, **haemorrhoids, jaundice, cyanosis, dropsy, amenorrhoea, haemorrhage** from the stomach, nose, lung, bladder and womb,**asthma, ulceration of lung, impotence, cataract, urinary calculus, paralysis, pain of thousands of kind**, etc."[72] are due to **psora**.

At the time of Hahnemann around 1800, medical science was not developed. Causative agent, pathogenesis, method of spread and prognosis of diseases were not known. That's why Hahnemann concluded wrongly that all chronic diseases are caused by only one agent—**psora**. Actually all diseases mentioned by Hahnemann have different causes. All students of biology and medical science know this fact. It is foolish to accept one cause for all diseases. Even today in Homeopathic colleges it is being taught.

12

If symptoms of disease are changed then drug should be changed.

ARGUMENT

Homeopathic treatment is based on the symptoms of disease. If symptoms are not produced then Homeopathy will not suggest any treatment. According to this pathy, if symptoms are not present then there is no treatment because drug is chosen only on the basis of similar symptoms produced in healthy person when drug is given.

In **hypertension**, in **early stage of cancer**, **open angle glaucoma**, and **diabetes**, there are no symptoms. Homeopathy will not suggest any treatment for these conditions. When diseases advance and conditions of patients deteriorate then only Homeopathy provides treatment due to presence of symptoms. In all those diseases where symptoms are not produced Homeopathy does not suggest any treatment.

Hahnemann writes— "During the treatment symptoms of disease should be studied. If symptoms are changed or new symptoms appear then drug should be changed."[73]

Homeopathy emphasized only on symptoms. There are various diseases in which at early stages symptoms are different than later stages. Examples of such diseases are **syphilis**, **tuberculosis**, **cancer**, **diabetes**, **glaucoma**.

According to Homeopathy, treatment at early stages will be different than treatment at later stages.

Treatments of **syphilis**, **diabetes**, **tuberculosis**, **cancer** are very specific irrespective of the stage of the disease. Same treatment is given, whether disease is at early stage or at advanced stage. So such importance given to symptoms by Homeopathy is absolutely wrong.

13

Hahnemann said— "It is only Homeopathy which can cure disease." Those who believe that there are other therapeutic methods also, do not know Homeopathy.

ARGUMENT

Hahnemann said— "It is impossible that there can be another true, best method of curing dynamic disease, besides Homeopathy. He who imagines that there are other modes of curing diseases besides it, could not have appreciated Homeopathy fundamentally nor practiced it with sufficient care, nor could he ever have seen or read cases of properly performed Homeopathic cures. My true, conscientious followers the pure Homeopathists, with their successful almost never failing treatment, might teach these persons better."[74]

Homeopathy says—"All other therapeutic methods are wrong" and supporters of Homeopathy should not use other therapeutic methods.

Then the government should discard modern medical science and Ayurveda from the society if it is really a supporter of Homeopathy. Followers of Homeopathy should never use modern medical science in their lifetime if they really are followers of Homeopathy.

14

All the curative power of medicines lies in the power of changing the state of man's health, and it is revealed by the observation of the latter. Hahnemann recommended drug of 30th potency for such studies.

ARGUMENT

Hahnemann writes— "'I was the first that opened up this path.' 'Business of a true physician relates to acquiring a knowledge of the instruments intended for the cure of the natural diseases investigating pathogenic power of the medicines, in order when called on to cure'. The whole pathogenic effect of the several medicines must be known, that is to say all the morbid symptoms and alteration in the health that each of them is specially capable of developing in the healthy individual must first have been observed as far as possible before we can hope to be able to find among them and toselect suitable Homeopathic remedies for most of the natural diseases."[75]

He also said— "Peculiar powers of medicines available for cure of disease are to be learned neither by any ingenious a prior speculations nor by the smell, taste, appearance of the drugs nor by their chemical analysis, nor yet by the employment of several of them at one time in a mixture (prescription) in diseases."[76]

Hahnemann had firm opinion that curative power of drug cannot be determined by studying them in patients. According to him a study (chemical or physical) of drugs is also useless.

If these concepts of determination of curative power of drugs are correct then all experimental studies should be stopped. Research and development of new drugs would be useless. According to Homeopathy, drug development is very easy. Administer a compound in a healthy individual and observe symptoms. That is sufficient. Hahnemann prescribed a method of studying curative power of drug in healthy human. "Medicinal substances are taken in high dilutions of **potentized** by proper **trituration** and **succussion** by which simple operations the powers which in their crude state lay hidden and as it were dormant, are developed and roused into activity to an incredible extent.... The plan we adopted is to give to the experimenter on an empty stomach, daily from four to six very small globules of the thirtieth potency of such a substance moistened with a little water or dissolved in more or less water and thoroughly mixed and let him continue this for several days."[77]

Hahnemann prescribed drug in 30th potency. Thirtieth potency means 1 in 10^{60} dilution. With this dilution, what I am saying is that there will not be any effect on human body because this concentration does not contain single molecule of a drug. By this dilution nothing can be observed. But what was observed by Hahnemann? He observed many pathological effects of drug in healthy body. If we observe and analyse minutely what was observed by Hahnemann was not accurate. His observations were false.

He writes—"Not all persons are affected by a medicine in an equally great degree; on the contrary there is a vast variety in this respect, so that sometimes an apparently weak individual may be scarcely at all affected by moderate dose of a medicine known to be of a powerful character whilst he is strongly enough acted on by others of a much weaker kind and on the other hand, there are very robust persons who experience very considerable morbid symptoms from an apparently mild medicine and only slight symptoms from a stronger drug."[78]

Hahnemann said during this study that sometimes severe morbid that symptoms are produced and sometimes by a similar drug only mild symptoms are developed.

He also said—"Among these symptoms, there occur in the case of some medicines not a few which are partially or under certain conditions directly opposite to other symptoms that have previously or subsequently appeared."[79]

"Subsequent dose often removes curatively some or the other symptoms caused by the previous dose or develops in its place an opposite state."[80]

He also writes— "All the symptoms, peculiar to a medicine do not appear in one person, nor all at once, nor in the same experiment but some occur in one person chiefly at one time, others again during a second or third trial, in another person some other symptoms appear but in such a manner that probably some of the phenomena are observed in the fourth, eighth, or tenth person which had already appeared in the second, sixth or ninth person and so forth; moreover they may not recur at the same hour."[81]

He also said— "It is very rare to develop all symptoms of a drug in a medium."[82] The above description indicates that there is no consistency in the development of symptoms by experimental drugs. There is a vast variety in this respect. Same dose sometimes produces strong symptoms and sometimes opposite symptoms. All symptoms of a drug are not produced in a single person. Different symptoms are produced in different persons at different times by different doses. It indicates that there is no uniformity and persistency in symptoms which should be there, if there is definite correlation between drug and symptoms. I am saying repeatedly that drug of such dilution cannot produce symptoms. Is it possible that symptoms can be produced without giving any drug just by suggestion? Yes. Study proved that symptoms can be produced without giving any drug. Studies have shown that "about 80 per cent of healthy people not taking any drug admit on questioning to symptoms (often several) such as commonly experienced as lesser adverse reactions to drugs." Therefore, to avoid misinterpretation these symptoms are intensified (or diminished) by administration of a placebo. Thus many symptoms may be wrongly attributed to drugs. There should be clear-cut and definite qualitative action of a drug in different subjects. For the definite amount of action minimum dose should be determined. Certainty and persistency in different subjects prove relation between drug and response. Minimum *pharmacological* effect will occur in all subjects when a certain amount of drug has been administered. Medical knowledge tells "augmented reaction will occur in everyone if enough of the drug is given because they are due to excess of normal predictable dose related to pharmacodynamic effects.'[84] With dilution of 30thpotency, uniform and persistent symptoms were not found by Hahnemann and studies also show that without prescribing drugs symptoms can be produced. We also know that drugs of this dilution contain no drug molecule. For the pharmacological action minimum amount of drug is necessary. Now we can say that the symptoms observed by Hahnemann with drugs of 30th potency were not related to drugs. It also means that the concept of Homeopathy regarding proving of drug by giving 30th potency is wrong. Even if the drug has been proved by giving it in concentrated form, this does not mean that this drug will be effective in diseases having similar **symptomatology**. And it is also true whendrug is given in Homeopathic doses, it has no curative effect.

Kent also writes—"Each prover takes a single dose of the medicine and wait to see if the single dose effect gives... . If we were attempting to prove a remedy like *silicate of alumina*, the master prover would advise the class not to interfere with the medicine for at least thirty days because its prodrome may be thirty days."[85] Here Kent advised for 30 days observation for proving of a drug. Pharmacokinetic knowledge is also important to get accurate conclusions. Orally giving drug in a single dose only cannot remain in gastrointestinal lumen for more than 48 hours. Either it will be absorbed from gastrointestine or it will pass out with stool. After absorption drug reaches the blood and then within an hour there will be onset of action. After that, metabolism and excretion starts. Peak effect on body diminishes gradually. Drugs may remain in body up to months but maximum peak effect will occur within a week, it cannot be delayed. Pharmacokinetic study means study regarding drug absorption, drug metabolism and excretion. Each drug has different pharmacokinetic character and its knowledge is a must to establish relation between drug and symptomatology it produces. If orally administered drug in single dose only produces action after seven days of its administration this indicates that such action has no relation with the orally administered drug. These symptoms must be due to some other cause or just psychological. Kent, Hahnemann and other Homeopaths made this mistake. Hahnemann and Kent never recommended study of Homeopathic drugs in patients. They recommended study of symptoms produced by drug in healthy bodies only. Now it is clear that the method used by Hahnemann and Kent for proving the drug is absolutely wrong.

15

Artificial disease produced by drug should be more powerful than natural disease then only it can displace pathological symptoms of disease.

ARGUMENT

Hahnemann defined primary and secondary actions. "Every agent acts upon the vitality, every medicine deranges more or less the vital force and causes a certain alteration in the health of the individual for a longer or shorter period. This is termed as primary action. To its action our vital force endeavors to oppose its own energy. This resistant action in a property is indeed an automatic action of our life preserving power, which goes by the name of secondary action or counter action." [86] Hahnemann has also written some examples of primary and secondary actions. "A hand bathed in hot water is at first much warmer than the other hand that has not been so treated (primary action); but when it is withdrawn from the hot water and again thoroughly dried it becomes in a short-time cold and at length much colder than the other (secondary action). A person heated by violent exercise (primary action) is afterwards affected with chills and shivering (secondary action). To one who was yesterday heated by drinking much wine (primary action), to-day every breath of air feels too cold (counteraction of the organism, secondary action). An arm that has been kept long in very cold water is at first much paler and colder (primary action) than the other, but removed from the cold water and dried, it subsequently becomes warmer, hot red."[87] This secondary action or counteraction is the reaction of the body against the primary action to maintain homeostasis. Body has capacity to maintain normal equilibrium in the body.

Hahnemann writes, accurately, "When a person falls ill, it is vital force everywhere present in his organism that is primarily deranged by the dynamic influence upon it of a morbific agent inimical to life; it is only the vital principle deranged to such an abnormal state, that can furnish the organism with its disagreeable sensations and incline it to the irregular process which we call disease."[88] "Vital force tries to control the diseases… . When causes of diseases are strong then only vital force does not suppress them and diseases are produced."[89] He also writes, "It is only the slighter and acute diseases that tend, when the natural period of their course has expired, to terminate quietly in resolution as it is called with or without the employment of not very aggressive allopathic remedies. The vital force having regained its power then gradually substitutes the normal condition for the derangement of the health that has now ceased to exist. But in severe acute and chronic diseases which constitute by far the greater portion of all the human ailments crude nature and the old school are equally powerless, in these neither the vital force with its self-aiding faculty, nor Allopathy in imitation of it."[90]

Hahnemann was right regarding this concept that vital power, natural capacity of body helps in fighting the disturbance of body and tries to maintain normal equilibrium. Today, we also know with our medical knowledge that "Normal cell function depends upon the constancy of this fluid, it is not surprising that in multicellular animals, an immense number of regulatory mechanisms have evolved to maintain it. To describe the various physiological arrangements which serve to restore the normal state, once it has been disturbed, W.B. Cannon coined the term homeostasis… . Many of these regulatory mechanisms operate on the principle of negative feedback, deviation from a given normal set point are detected by a sensor, and signals from the sensor trigger compensatory changes that continue until the set point is again reached."[91]

"As long as normal conditions are maintained in this internal environment, the cells of the body continue to live and function properly. Extreme dysfunction leads to death whereas moderate dysfunction leads to sickness."[92]

Hahnemann emphasises the curative power of vital force. Slighter and acute diseases are resolved spontaneously. He said that if disturbing agents are of shorter duration, then they can be controlled easily by compensatory mechanism of body. When homoeostasis fails, disease starts. Symptomatology of disease develops only when homoeostasis has failed.

Hahnemann said, "A weaker dynamic affection is permanently extinguished in the living organism by a stronger one, if the latter (whilst differing in kind) is very similar to the former in its manifestations."[93] "The curative power of medicines, therefore, dependson their symptoms similar to the disease but superior to it in strength. So that eachindividual case of disease is most surely radically, rapidly and permanently annihilated and removed only by a medicine capable of producing (in the human system) in the most similar and complete manner the totality of its symptoms which at the same time are stronger than the disease."[94]

Here Hahnemann wanted to say that natural disease can be cured by Homeopathic drug which produces symptoms as produced by disease. Here Hahnemann was wrong. Disease already has disturbed homoeostasis. Similar symptoms if produced by drug will further disturb the homoeostasis. Then vital force of body cannot compensate. Homeopathic drug, by creating similar symptomatology, willdeteriorate vital capacity of body further. Disease cannot be cured by this method. Actually Homeopathic drugs used in such dilutions can never produce symptoms in a healthy body. If Homeopathic drugs produce symptoms in healthy body, disease will be aggravated definitely. For example "*leptazole* is a compound that is commonly used toproduce convulsion. It is usually injected subcutaneously as 1 per cent solution is needed in the dose of 100 mg/kg body weight."[95] It will be impossible to cure an **epileptic patient** by giving *leptazole* in such doses that produces convulsion. There will be death in place of cure if *leptazole* is given during convulsion. Similarly, we can say that by this mechanism diseases cannot be cured, they are only aggravated. According to Hahnemann, *leptazole* will be the best drug in epilepsy when given in 30th potency, but things are not like this. Discovery of drug is not so simple. Hahnemann was wrong. He also did not explain how pathological symptoms can cure the disease of similar symptoms. He knew his limitations, that's why he writes—"It matters little what may be the scientific explanation of how it takes place and I do not attach much importance to the attempts made to explain it."[96] His arguments in this favour are ridiculous. "The stronger disease, namely, annihilates the weaker and that for simple reason, because of the stronger morbific power. When it invades the system by reason of its similarity of action, involves precisely the same parts of the organism that were previously affected by the weaker morbid imitation, which consequently can no longer act on these parts, but is extinguished just as the image of lamp's flame is rapidly overpowered and effaced from our retina by thestronger sunbeam impinging on the eye."[97]

Such philosophical arguments have no place in science.

Regarding this matter Hahnemann was confused that's why he made contradictory statements. At one place he writes—"Artificial disease produced by Homeopathic drug is more powerful than natural disease."[98] "According to nature, disease can be removed solely by one that is similar in symptoms and is somewhat stronger."[99]

In another place Hahnemann writes, "In Homeopathic cure, after the destruction of natural disease a certain amount of medicinal disease remains in the organism but on account of the extra minuteness of the dose it is so transient, so slight and disappears so rapidly of its own accord, that the vital force has no need to employ against this small artificial derangement of its health."[100]

Hahnemann writes at one place that artificial symptoms produced by Homeopathic drug are stronger and powerful than natural disease, while at another place he writes that during Homeopathic treatment the extraordinary minuteness of the dose of Homeopathic drug produces transient and slight symptoms that disappear spontaneously.

Hahnemann did not explain cause of this contradiction. He mentioned only, "After destruction of natural disease symptoms produced by Homeopathic drugs become very mild."[101]

How does it take place? What is the logic behind this comment? Nothing has been said by him. At one place Hahnemann writes, "Excessively minute dose requisite for Homeopathic use is too weak to produce the other symptoms of the medicine that are not Homeopathic in case of those parts of the body that are free from disease."[102]

Hahnemann said that Homeopathic drug has no effect on healthy organs. It acts only on diseased organs having pathological symptoms. And in proving of drug he writes that Homeopathic drugs produce symptoms in healthy organs of healthy body when given in 30th potency. Again there is a contradiction of the use of a very minute quantity of drug. If Homeopathic drug produces symptoms in healthy organs of healthy human beingthen it should produce symptoms in healthy organs of patients. But he denied it.

At one point, Hahnemann writes that after destruction of natural disease, remaining morbid symptoms of drug in the body "disappear so rapidly of its own accord that the vital force has no need to employ"[103] and "when natural disease has been removed vital force does not require to do any effort to abolish the remaining drug induced symptoms".[104] At another place he writes—"After removal of natural disease drug induced symptoms of short duration are abolished by vital force"[105] and "In the Homeopathic curative operation the living organism reacts from these only so much as is requisite to raise the health again to the normal healthy state"[106] and "vital force uses its power against drug induced effect".[107] That indicates Hahnemann himself was not clear. There are many contradictions in explanations given by him.

Hahnemann said that symptoms produced by drug should be more powerful and stronger than similar symptoms of disease then only cure is possible. Because powerful and strong symptoms of drug only replace comparatively weaker and similar symptoms of disease. This indicates that a patient suffering from pain in abdomen can get cured only by that Homeopathic drug which can create more severe pain in abdomen. A Homeopathic drug should develop more intense headache in a patient who is suffering from headache then only will the drug be effective. It cannot be possible for a drug to cure a disease by producing same symptoms as produced by disease itself. It will rather aggravate the problem.

16

Mercuric chloride is effective in very dilute concentration and its toxic effect is similar as symptomatology of **syphilis**. It is according to the rules of Homeopathy.

ARGUMENT

Hahnemann made an important law of Homeopathy *like cures like*, by observation of *cinchona* and *mercury*. **Cinchona** was used in **malaria** and *mercury* was used in **syphilis**.

"Hahnemann had been impressed with the particular symptoms which mercury could produce and had associated these with its healing capacities in **syphilis**."[108] That's why his conclusion was "Displacing a disease by similar medicine which could cause similar states to those which it could cure."[109]

It has already been explained earlier how Hahnemann concluded wrongly by observing *cinchona* effect in **malaria** and in a healthy human being. Now, it is being explained how Hahnemann was misled by mercury. "Many chemicals are toxic to cell protoplasm. In certain instances they may possess a specific affinity and toxicity for micro-organisms of a special type *e.g. antimalarial drugs*. In other cases, the effect upon cells may be non-selective and cells of the host as well as invading bacteria may be killed. Protoplasmic poison (*mercury salts* and *silver salts*) belong to the latter category. For this reason, these agents must be used judiciously as antiseptic."[110]

"The metal acts in extremely low concentration if allowed sufficient time. *Mercuric chloride* kills B. Typhosus at dilution of 1 in 10,00,000 in 24 hours and at a dilution of 1 in 20,000 in 22 minutes."[111] "*Mercury* was the first drug effective in the treatment of **syphilis**."[112]

"Like other *mercury salts*, *mercuric chloride* has a specific toxic action against Trepanoma pallidium and has been used in the treatment of **syphilis**."[113]

"*Mercury* is highly toxic to body. 1 to 5 μg/ml concentration of *mercury* in blood produces various toxic manifestations.**Acute mercury poisoning** is characterized by ashen grey appearance of the mouth, pharynx, and gastric mucosa, vomiting, diarrhoea, emphysema, haemorrhage. Kidney, colon and mouth are also affected. Renal lesions are also produced. In **chronic mercury poisoning** features are **paraesthesias,** ataxia, visual defects, **dysarthria**, hearing defects, tremors, and various neurological and psychiatric symptoms. Irritability, erethism, insomnia, confusion, forgetfulness are common psychiatric symptoms of **chronic mercury poisoning**. **Nephrotoxicity,** gingivitis, **stomatitis** and other non-specific symptoms like anorexia, weight loss, anemia, and weakness are also associated with chronic mercury poisoning."[114]

The **symptomatology** of **syphilis** is more or less **akin to** mercury toxic manifestations. "**Syphilis** is a chronic systemic infection caused by trepanoma pallidium, a spirochaete (a micro-organism).**Syphilis** has wide symptomatology. These are macular papular, papulosquamous skin rashes; mucosa erosions in lips, oral mucosal, tongue palate, pharynx, vulva, vagina; silver grey erosive mucosal patches surrounded by red periphery; fever, weight loss, malaise, anorexia, gasteritis, **hepatitis**, **nephropathy**. **Arthritis**, ocular disturbances, **optic neuritis**, ataxia, paraesthesias, bladder disturbances,abnormalities regarding personality, illusion, delusion, hallucination, alteration on intellect functions. Renal involvement is associated with proteinuria, an **acute nephritic syndrome** or with haemorrhage."[115]

Now, by observing and comparing **mercury toxicity** and **syphilis** manifestation, we can say both are more or less similar. But with this similarity 'the rule' *like cures like*, cannot be formulated. Observation of Hahnemann was correct but the conclusion was wrong. Why?

"*Mercury* and its compounds are absorbed through the skin, by ingestion and by inhalation. Inorganic compounds of *mercury* are absorbed through the gastrointestinal tract better than the organic oxidized and the mercury salts form soluble compounds with proteins, sodium chloride, blood and tissue fluid alkalis... . Mercury inhibits enzyme system and disturb mitochondrial functions, it also combines with sulfhydryl and phosphoryl group in the cell membrane."[116]

"Infection in **syphilis** occurs by penetration of the spirochaetes through a microscopic break in epithelial lining of the mucosa or the skin into connective tissue. There they rapidly multiply, penetrate the lymphatics and invade the blood stream producing a systemic spirochetemia... . This organism may produce extensive tissue necrosis involving all tissues of the body."[117]

Mercury produces various toxic manifestations because *mercury* damages cells and ultimately tissues of various organs of body. Spirochaetes, causative organism in **syphilis** also produce more or less similar symptomatology because it also damages various organs of the body. *Mercury* has non-specific action. It destroys human cells as well as foreign micro-organisms which may be spirochaetes or bacteria. The concentration of *mercury* which is required to kill spirochaetes also destroys human cells. *Mercury* also destroys bacteria and it is also effective as antibacterial and antiseptic. In various bacterial infections, mercury is effective but these bacterial infections like B typhosus never produce *symptomatology* like mercury-toxic manifestations. This finding is against the law discovered by Hahnemann. *Mercury* is effective in very low concentration. This misled Hahnemann that drugs could be effective in very low concentration.

It is by chance that *mercury* and T. pallidium, both have common pathogenesis for producing toxic effects in human body. But by this observation generalization cannot be made. Today, *mercury* is not used in systemic infections due to toxic manifestations.

Penicillin is the drug of choice for **syphilis**. When *penicillin* is administered in healthy human being it never produces **syphilis** like symptomatology. It again goes against Hahnemann.

17

Hahnemann observed the effect of opium on human beings and saw two types of effects direct and indirect. Both were opposite to each other. He said that first direct action was initial aggravation of symptoms. Similar effect was also seen when sulphur had been given to treat skin diseases.

ARGUMENT

Hahnemann observed in his practice that medicine has two types of actions, direct and indirect. He gives the example of *opium*. "This drug at first produces a fearless elevation of spirit, a sensation of strength and high courage, an imaginative gaiety. But after some hours have passed we find the person so elevated as a first result of taking the drug relaxed, dejected, peevish with confused memory and generally discomforted and fearful."[118] The first action is direct action and secondary action is indirect action.

"Hahnemann welcomed first action with some accentuation of the patient symptoms. The secondary or indirect action were decided in favour of reduction in the symptoms and in cure."[119]

Initial aggravation of symptoms by *opium* was called first action of drug and on this basis Hahnemann made another concept of Homeopathy.

By this observation Hahnemann made another false concept of Homeopathy as he writes:

"The slight homeopathic aggravation during the first hour—a very good prognostic that the acute disease will most probably yield to the first dose—is quite as it right to be."[120]

Cause of this aggravation was given by Hahnemann as follows:

"Immediately after ingestion—for the first hour or for a few hours causes a kind of slight aggravation when the dose as not be insufficiently small which has so much resemblance to the original disease that it seems to the patient to be an aggravation of his own disease. But it is in reality nothing more than an extremely similar medicinal disease, somewhat exceeding in strength of the original affection."[121]

Hahnemann suggested that this aggravation of symptoms is due to similar symptomatology produced by drug in addition to symptoms produced by disease. This suggestion was made on the basis of effect produced by opium in healthy body. Here again Hahnemann made wrong conclusion. How? *Opium* and its derivatives are drugs of addiction. "With therapeutic doses,*morphine* (*opium* derivatives) produces a sense of emotional well being or contentment termed euphoria. Euphoria eliminates the normal fear, panic, withdrawal and flight response to pain and aids the analgesic action of *morphine.* The ability to produce euphoria even in the absence of pain makes *morphine* one of the worst drugs of addiction."[122]

The euphoric effect produced by *opium* confused Hahnemann who later on framed wrong Homeopathic concepts of aggravation of symptoms by Homeopathic drugs.

Euphoria means false sense of well being, produced by *opium*. This effect confused Hahnemann. He correlated this euphoriatic effect with aggravation of disease symptom wrongly. I am writing again and again that single or few observations do notmake any conclusion. There should be controlled experiments by proper expert then only conclusion can be drawn.

The exaltation of the medicinal symptoms are also observed by other physicians when by accident they prescribed Homeopathic remedy. "When a patient suffering fromitch complains so an increase of the eruption after sulfur, his physician who knows not the cause of this consoles him with the assurance that the itch must first come outproperly before it can be cured."[123]

Sulphur is used in skin infection. "*Sulphur* is converted into *pentathionic* acid in order to exert germicidal action. *Sulfur* also possess a Keratolytic property which may be the basis for the therapeutic action of the element in certain cutaneous disorder... . Sulfur is used as a fungicide and parasiticide. It is widely used in treatment of the **cutaneous** disorders such as **prolonged seborrhea** and **eczema dermatitis**. Prolonged local use of sulphur may result in characteristic **dermatitis venenata**."[124] It is an acute **allergic inflammation** of the skin caused by contact with sulphur.

Again, we can conclude that exaltation of itch is actually sulphur eruption that assumes the appearance of an increase of the itch. This fact was not known to these physicians, that's why they arrived at wrong conclusions and made wrong generalisations. These actions of *opium* and sulphur are very specific and on this basis a general rule cannot be made.

18

About the year 1500... Melampus, a most celebrated physician, is said to have cured the daughters of Proteus...who were affected by **wandering mania**, they were cured chiefly by means of *veratrum album*.... As the plant could also cause mania, the story was of two-fold interest to Hahnemann.

ARGUMENT

In support of Hahnemann's law of similarity examples were given from the history. "About the year 1500 **Melampus**, ... a most celebrated physician, is said to have cured the daughters of Proteus... who were affected by a **wandering mania**, they were cured chiefly by means of *veratrum album*, given in the milk of goats fed upon **veratrum**. As the plant could also cause **mania**, the story was of two-fold interest to Hahnemann."[125]

In this example two things are important. First, *veratrum* cured *mania* and second, *veratrum* produced *mania*. This example supported Hahnemann's law of similarity.

To assess the effect of a drug, we should know what is the normal course of a disease when we are not giving any treatment. Knowledge of natural course of a disease is very very important in the absence of treatment. To study the effect of a drug three groups of patients are usually made. Each group consists of a large number of patients according to study material. Drug is given to one group. For second group drug is not given, and for third group inert material is given for treatment to see placebo (psychological) effect. Only by statistical analysis conclusion can be drawn. By observing only one or few patients without systematic controlled study nothing can be said.

If by study we find that in natural course, without taking any drug a disease subsides automatically then without doing any controlled clinical study how can we say that disease is cured by taking a drug. For example, **bacillary dysentery** is cured automatically within 24 hours without taking any treatment. If we give any treatment to this patient, it will seem to be effective. But it will not be the truth. It will be the false conclusion. Similarly **manic** episode subsides automatically and after a period of normalcy again there is an episode of **manic reaction**. It is a normal cycle for manic patient that first there is **mania** then **normalcy** and after sometime again there is mania. It has been mentioned in psychiatry.

Maniac depressive reactions tend to be episodic and relatively brief. Even in those cases where no formal treatment is received, **manic reactions** usually run their course in about three months and **depressive reactions** in about nine months. There are wide variations, however, with some psychotic episodes lasting only a few days and others as long as a year or more. At the conclusion of a **manic** or **depressive episode**, the individual usually returns to apparent normalcy."[126]

It is also mentioned in psychiatry that "Duration of episodes in the pre-drug era averaged about one year for **depression** and four months for **mania**. Patients who present with only symptoms of **depression** take almost twice as long to recover from their episode (a median of 9 weeks) as do patients present with only symptoms of **mania** (a median of 5 weeks). Short-term recovery rates also differ among subtypes. Bipolar patients, however, are more likely than unipolar patients to have multiple subsequent episodes."[127] By above discussion we can conclude that in **manic-patients** Hahnemann observed wrongly that by giving *veratrum*, patient is improving and by giving *veratrum* patient gets attack of mania. Second point in favour of our argument is that *veratrum* alkaloid does not produce any psychological and neurological effect when given to healthy persons. Hahnemann observed attack of mania in these patients after giving *veratrum* who were already suffering from mania. Once a patient has been suffered from mania there are chances that he will again get an episode of mania. It is a normal cycle. He concluded wrongly that it was *veratrum* which is responsible for recurrence of manic episodes. *Veratrum* has no psychological effect. "On oral administration 1 to 25 mg. daily in divided doses is effective in lowering the blood pressure in about one-third of the patients with hypertension. Unless dosage is regulated carefully toxic effects such as nausea, vomiting, hiccough, severe hypotension, **bradycardia** or even heart block appear."[128]

Thus, I would like to conclude that*veratrum* does not cause mania or depression.

19

Hahnemann recommended *belladonna* for treatment of scarlet fever in an infinitesimal dose because it produces fever. In 1838, the Persian Government ordered doctors to use *belladonna* in small doses against the epidemics of scarlet fever because it was effective. It supported Hahnemann's rule—"like cures like."

ARGUMENT

Treatment of **scarlet fever** by *belladonna* also created confusion in the mind of Hahnemann.

"Hahnemann recommended on the ground of it being a similar was *belladonna* for **scarlet fever**. This medicine moreover he administered in a very high potency, that is in an **infinitesimal** dose."[129]

Hahnemann writes—"me with no remedy so capable of producing a counterpart if the symptoms here present as *belladonna*. I, therefore, gave this to a girl of 10 years of age, who was already affected by the first stage of **scarlet fever**, a dose of this medicine 1/432999th part of a grain of the extract, which according to my subsequent experience is rather too large a dose. So remarkable was the effect that the following day she was playing again, complaining of nothing and quite lively."[130]

This observation compelled Hahnemann to think regarding preventive aspect of *belladonna* in **scarlet fever**.

"The doctor then recollected that some weeks before he had visited a family where three children lay sicken with **scarlet fever**, the eldest daughter alone, who had been taking *belladonna* not having sickened. And this although during previous epidemics the eldest daughter had shown a disposition to take them first. He straightaway, therefore gave *belladonna* to the remaining five children of the family. He was now, giving very small doses of the drug every 72 hours and they all remained well throughout the epidemics."[131]

"In 1838, Persian Government ordered the doctors of the country to use *belladonna* in small doses against the epidemics of **scarlet fever**."[132]

However, some physicians had opposed Hahnemann by saying about the "smallness of the dose". It was also stated that powder contained no *belladonna*. But it had been established at that time that belladonna was effective in **scarlet fever**, as a curative and as a preventive drug.

Now, we are analyzing treatment of **scarlet fever** by *belladonna*. *Belladonna* produces fever in healthy individuals and *belladonna* is effective in **scarlet fever** as told by Hahnemann and which also supported the law of similar, framed by Hahnemann. Today we know that—"The *belladonna* drugs are widely distributed in nature especially in the solanaceae plants. *Atropa belladonna* yields mainly the alkaloid *atropine*. The rise in body temperature due to the *belladonna alkaloids* is usually significant only after large doses. Nevertheless in infants and small children moderate doses induce atropine fever. Suppression of sweating is without doubt a considerable factor in the production of the fevers, animals that do not sweat such as the dogs do not exhibit fever after *atropine*."[133]

The observation of Hahnemann that *belladonna* increases the temperature of the body was correct. Today we know the mechanism how *belladonna* increases body temperature. Suppression of sweating is mainly responsible for pyrexia. Second part of this observation that *belladonna* is effective in **scarlet fever** was wrong.

Now, it is known by pathological study and normal prognosis of the disease that, "It became apparent that only a minority of adults were susceptible to **scarlet fever** and that the number who were immune was far in excess to the number who had actually had the disease previously. It appears that repeated experiences with **streptococcus pyogenes** may confer immunity to **scarlet fever** even though the disease, per se, has not been experienced. The importance of individual variation in the host is illustrated by the fact that several or all members of a family may develop **streptococcal pharyngitis** from the same strain of organism, yet only one of the group may develop **scarlet fever** the other manifesting only **nasopharyngitis**."[134] We should also understand this fact that

$$\text{"Severity of disease} = \frac{\text{Virulence of bacteria} \times \text{Number/Portal of entry"}}{\text{Resistance of host}}.$$[135]

It means if micro-organism is virulent and size of infecting dose is high, the disease will be severe and in opposite conditions disease will be mild. Similarly, host resistance also plays an important role. If host resistance is high disease will be mild and if host resistance is poor disease will be severe. This rule is true for all bacterial, viral and other infections. "Variation in host resistance are often the result of variation in the host's ability to form antibody."[136]

Now we can conclude that intensity of**scarlet fever** will be mild if host resistance is high or infecting organism has low virulence and low doses. During observation of **scarlet fever** it has been found that—

"**Scarlet fever** has many varieties. In the mild type, the patient never appears particularly ill. Toxaemia is negligible, the temperature does not exceed 38.3°C (101°F) and symptomatic recovery takes place, within three to four days. This type of **scarlet fever** covers larger per cent of cases. In more severe cases, the **prodromal** symptoms are more striking with the temperature reaching 104°F, the rash heavier and lasting for a few days while fever and constitutional symptoms may persist up to a week. Complications are more common to this group."[137]

Now we can understand very well where Hahnemann committed the mistake.

Hahnemann cured a patient of **scarlet fever** who had been suffering from first stage of **scarlet fever**. Actually this patient had been suffering from mild **scarlet fever**. The cure was automatic and mild **scarlet fever** has a very short course. During automaticrecovery of mild **scarlet fever** Hahnemann administered *belladonna* and concluded wrongly that the fever was cured due to *belladonna*. Hahnemann did not know that mild type of **scarlet fever** recovers early. It has been mentioned in reference no. 131 that the eldest daughter who had been taking *belladonna* did not suffer from **scarlet fever** and they also mentioned that this eldest daughter had suffered from **scarlet fever** in previous years. Today we know that if a person suffers from**scarlet fever** he develops immunity to **scarlet fever** then he will never develop this disease in next infections. This fact was not previously known. That's why they derived wrong conclusion. They did not understand that this elder daughter had suffered from **scarlet fever** earlier so she could not have suffered from **scarlet fever** in the coming years due to immunity. The immunity of the eldest daughter to scarlet fever was not related to *belladonna* in anyway.

Hahnemann has mentioned in reference no. 131 that children, who were taking *belladonna* did not suffer from **scarlet fever** because of *belladonna*. It is also wrong. We know by present study as written in reference no. 105 that it is not necessary that all members of family should suffer from **scarlet fever** during epidemics. Some may suffer from **pharyngitis** only to give immunity to **scarlet fever**. It has been studied during epidemics that only few members of family suffered from **scarlet fever**, remaining members remain healthy without giving *belladonna* or any other treatment. So, this is the truth that *belladonna* has no preventive and curative role in the **scarlet fever**.

Again this origin of Homeopathic concept is wrong.

To know the effect of a treatment it should be compared with normal course of a disease. And it should be clear in the mind of all the readers that normal observations are normal observations. These observations are part of present medical science. Without observing a disease nothing can be said regarding treatment. Various misconceptions are prevalent in the society due to lack of scientific studies in the field of medicine. For example, many unscientific therapies claim treatment of **warts** but the fact is —

"**Wart** is due to virus and is infectious. As **warts** often disappear spontaneously, any treatment which is in use at the time will gain an undeserved reputation as a **wart** cure."[138]

20

Clinical experience proved that the medicinal virtues were undoubtedly increased by the process of attenuation, trituration and succussion. By **dilution** and **trituration** effects of *mercury* and *arsenic* are increased. By grinding, insoluble substances become soluble and give colours that also supports the view that dilution increases power.

ARGUMENT

One of the main concepts of Homeopathy ispotentisation. Potentisation means increased potency by dilution and **trituration**. Homeopaths say "As clinical experience proved that the medicinal virtues were undoubtedly increased by the process of attenuation, **trituration** and succussion, Hahnemann called those process potentisation, that is making more potent for cure though less powerful for harm."[139]

Hahnemann also wrote—"Pure *gold*, *silver*, *platinum* have no action on the health in their solid state nor crude vegetable, charcoal, etc. These substances are in a state of suspended animation as regards the medicinal action, but triturate one grain of **gold** leaf with 100 grains of sugar of milk and a preparation results which has already great medicinal power."[140]

By **dilution** and **trituration** the effect of *mercury* is increased. But this potentisation is not due to dilute *mercury* but it is due to the formation of mercuric oxide which is highly potent in higher dilution than concentrated mercury. We know this by the knowledge of chemistry.

"*Silver* undergoes no change in water or pure air. *Silver* is unaffected by caustic alkalis even on fusion and by vegetable acids. Dilute hydrochloric acid and sulphuric acid also have no action."[141]

"*Gold* does not tarnish when exposed to air or oxygen even at high temperature. Common acids do not attack it if they are used one by one."[142]

"*Platinum* is a noble metal and is very slightly affected even on prolonged heating in air. It is very resistant to the action of acids. Boiling concentrated sulphuric acid attacks it to a slight extent."[143]

Above reference nos. 141, 142 and 143 from chemistry show that *silver*, *gold* and *platinum* metals after dilution and **trituration** do not modify into other compounds because these are highly resistant to air, water and acid. Whereas *mercury* as well as *arsenic* change into other compounds after **trituration** and dilution which are highly potent than original metals. As we know about arsenic that "Metallic *arsenic* is not poisonous as it is insoluble in water and, therefore incapable of absorption from the alimentary canal but it oxidizes by exposure to the air and then becomes poisonous. It is believed that some portion of elementary *arsenic* may undergo oxidation in the alimentary canal and some conditions may produce poisonous symptoms."[144]

By the knowledge of chemistry we also know that "when *arsenic* is burnt in air, Arsenous oxide is produced which acts as a violent irritant poison."[145]

With the help of the above information, we can conclude that mercury and *arsenic* gave wrong impressions to Hahnemann. Hahnemann thought wrongly about *mercury* and *arsenic*. *Mercury* and *arsenic* in their original metallic form were not potent but after **dilution** and **trituration** these were converted into other compounds as they become potent and toxic in dilute forms and effective in some diseases but highly toxic. Hahnemann's conclusions regarding **silver**, **gold** and **platinum** were wrong. These metals after dilution and trituration never become potent. They are not effective in medicine in their original metallic form. These metals in high dilution have no effect in any disease.

Today, compounds of *mercury* and *arsenic* are not used as a drug because these are highly toxic even in high dilutions. But *mercury* and *arsenic* give wrong foundation to Homeopathy because these metals after **dilution** and **trituration** convert into potent compounds. These observations made wrong law of Homeopathy that **dilution** and **trituration** increase potency of a substance. Supporters of Homeopathy also give examples of colloids by mistake. They thought by grinding down insoluble substances, solutions are made which give colours. These colours represent hidden power of substances. It has been said that by grinding insoluble substances they became soluble which represent increase in medicinal power. Hahnemann supported "grinding of *gold* for medicinal purposes finely enough to pass into something approaching a soluble state."[146]

Homeopaths took support ofCennino. "Cennino left his directions for the preparation of vegetable and mineral substances for use in painting of pictures explaining how by various degree of pulverisation their peculiar beauties could be released of the blue made from grinding lapis lazuli to a powder. Cennino told it as noble, beautiful and perfect beyond all other colours."[147] "By grinding, insoluble substances become soluble and give colours. It is due to formation of Colloids."[148]

If sand is shaken with water it results suspension. Due to large size, the sand particles would settle down on standing. If particle size is reduced gradually then at the size of 1 to 100 nm colloidal state is formed. In this condition solution appears homogenous and particles do not settle down on standing. Particles are not separable by ordinary filtration. Coarser particles are broken to the colloidal size by grinding and colour of the colloidal solution depends upon (1) Size and shape of particles, (2) Wavelength of the light passing through the solution, (3) Selective absorption power of solution, (4) Observer receives the light by transmission or reflection. Conclusively it can be said— "Colloidal state does not indicate class of substances but is a state. Any substance can be brought into colloidal state."

Hahnemann did not know about colloids that's why he wrongly interpreted this state. Not only *gold* but any substance can be transformed into colloidal state. In this state substance gives colour and becomes soluble. This stage depends upon particle size and does not give any extra medicinal capacity to that substance.

21

Allopathic treatment was unscientific, wrong and responsible for more harm than cure. Hahnemann opposed Allopathy and established Homeopathy. One prescription of Hahnemann which made him very popular was treatment of **Cholera**. Allopathy was not able to cure the patients of cholera but Homeopathy did it.

ARGUMENT

I am saying repeatedly that Allopathy treatment prevalent at the time of Hahnemann was unscientific, wrong and responsible for more harm than cure. This treatment was totally different from Allopathy of the present day which is absolutely scientific and based on practical knowledge.

Here is one more example of old Allopathy treatment. "Nervous attack from early childhood was treated by Moxa and trephine. **Moxa** was a cylinder of readily combustible material which is burnt on the skin. Trephine means removal of a part of the bone of the skull."[149] Old Allopathy treatment of Hahnemann's time was harmful. Homeopathic treatment was actually no treatment. No treatment is always better than harmful treatment. Harmful treatment damages the body while no treatment does not interfere the immunity of body which is helpful in fighting the disease. One more example is being given here:

"One doctor Lagusius had admittedly tried to fight the severe fever and its accompanying symptoms by venesection and when this failed to give relief he proceeded to open the veins again and again until blood-letting had been resorted to for a fourth time... . To abstract the fluid of life four times in 24 hours from a man who has lost flesh from mental overwork combined with a long continued **diarrhoea** without procuring any improvement."[150]

One prescription of Hahnemann which made him very popular was treatment of **cholera**. In this prescription *camphor* was directed to the arresting of **cholera**. "Hahnemann had not treated or even seen one single **cholera** patient. Hahnemann had procured a very accurate description of the symptoms and had found that the first and most important of these in **cholera** patient resembled one another and were similar to the symptoms produced if *camphor* was taken in large quantities by a healthy individual."[151]

Here, one thing should be clear that to study the symptoms of a drug produced in healthy individual, drug has been given in large amount.

When camphor is given in large amount it produces symptomatology similar to **cholera** because *camphor* is an irritant substance to gastrointestinal tract. "Hahnemann had, therefore, concluded from the great similarity of the symptoms at the beginning of the disease with those brought out by *camphor* in the proving that this ought to be the best remedy to give at the outset. Similarly, he also prescribed the other remedies required for the cure of the later stages of **cholera**."[152] According to Hahnemann, at an early stage of **cholera** camphor in high dilution is effective but in later stage of **cholera** other drugs are effective. By this treatment Hahnemann had become very popular. "In 1854, a report to the House of Commons gave the figures of death from **cholera** under orthodox treatment at 59.2 per cent and under the Homeopathic treatment at 16.4 per cent. In all 54,000 persons died."[153]

By the success of this **cholera** treatment, Homeopathy became very popular throughout the world.

But it was the wrong popularity of Homeopathic treatment. The fact is that "**Cholera** is an acute **diarrhoea** disease caused by **vibrio cholerae** OL classical or EL TOR. Epidemiological studies have shown that more than 90 per cent of classical **cholera** cases are mild and clinically indistinguishable from other acute**diarrhoeas**. A typical case of **cholera** shows three stages. First stage is of evacuation characterized by profuse painless watery **diarrhoea** followed by vomiting. The patient soon passes into a stage of collapse because of dehydration. Death may occur at this stage due to dehydration and acidosis resulting from**diarrhoea.** If death does not occur the patient begins to show signs of clinical improvement. The classical form of severe **cholera** occurs in only 5 to 10 per cent of cases. In the rest, the disease tends to be mild characterized by**diarrhoea** with or without vomiting or marked dehydration. As a rule mild cases recover in one to three days."[154]

When treatment of **cholera** is considered it is mentioned clearly in the text book of medicine that "the disease runs its course in two to seven days and subsequent manifestations depend on the adequacy of electrolyte repletion therapy. With prompt fluid and electrolyte repletion, physiological recovery is remarkable, rapid and mortality is exceptionally rare under ideal conditions and with prompt and adequate fluid replacement, mortality approacheszero."[155]

By studying reference nos. 151 to 155, we can compare Homeopathic treatment of cholera with old Allopathic orthodox treatment and with new Allopathic medicine treatment. With the help of modern medical treatment death rate in **cholera** is zero. There is no death if modern allopathic treatment is given. This indicates there is 100 per cent cure rate.

We also know that 90 per cent **cholera** cases are mild and recover automatically within one to three days. There is 10 per cent death rate in **cholera** if no treatment is given. WhenHomeopathic treatment has been given there is death rate of 16.4 per cent. Death rate duringHomeopathic treatment is same as when any type of treatment is not given. This indicates Homeopathy treatment is equal to no treatment in **cholera** patients.

By old orthodox Allopathic treatment in **cholera**, there is a death rate of 59.2 per cent. When treatment is not given there is a death rate of 10 per cent only. This suggests that there is a damaging influence of old orthodox treatment in **cholera**, and this is correct. "Medicine as commonly practiced in Allopathy knows no treatment except todraw from diseases the injurious materials which are assumed to be their cause. The blood of the patient is made to flow, mercilessly by bleeding ... medicine as commonly practiced seek to evacuate the contents of the stomach and sweep the intestine clearly of the materials assumed to originate diseases."[156] Medicine employed in **cholera** in orthodox allopathic treatment increases blood loss and water loss. In**cholera**, there is already dehydration which is further increased by old Allopathic treatment. That's why there is increased death rate by old Allopathic treatment.

Now we can conclude that old Allopathic treatment of**cholera** is worst. Homeopathic treatment is no treatment while modern Allopathic treatment is accurate treatment and gives 100 per cent cure rate.

22

According to Homeopathy, causes of diseases are actually inside the body, not outside. Bacteria, viruses, protozoa, mosquito, dirty water, unhygienic food and pollution are not responsible for any disease. The basic cause of all diseases is **psora** and that is developed due to wrong thoughts. Sinful thoughts and sinful acts are responsible for all chronic diseases. If a person has pure thought, he cannot suffer from any disease.

ARGUMENT

"Homeopathy says it is useless to expend money in discovering cause of diseases. Government is expending lacs of rupees unnecessarily in such studies. Why this truth cannot be accepted by people that the cause of disease is actually inside the body not outside the body."[157]

Do you accept this statement of Homeopathy? Development of medical science is not only dependent on medical research but it is also related to total development of science. Invention of the microscope in physics is responsible for discovery of bacteria and virus. In the absence of microscope, it was not possible to search bacteria and virus. Discovery of bacteria and virus with this study holds these organisms responsible for diseases and give tremendous help to medical science. Medical science is taking help from physics, chemistry, botany, zoology biotechnology, genetics. Concepts of medical science are based on various branches of science. By study we know today "**Malaria** is a protozoal disease caused by parasites of the genus plasmodium and transmitted to man by certain species of infected female Anophelese mosquito." Ronald Ross discovered the transmission of malaria by **Anophelese** mosquito in 1897. Ross found **malarial** parasites grow as cyst on the stomach wall of an Anophelese mosquito. Killing mosquito by D.D.T. and destroying malarial parasite by **anti-malarial** drugs ensured that **malaria** came down to extremely low levels. We know all these facts then how can we accept thisconcept of Homeopathy that malaria is not caused by malarial parasite. Similarly in Homeopathy, killing of parasite and killing of mosquito are not required in the treatment of **malaria**.

"According to Homeopathy the basic cause of all diseases is **psora.** If no **psora** is in the body, there cannot be any disease. This **psora** is developed due to wrong thoughts and can transfered from generations to generations."[158] **Psora** expresses itself by skin disease associated with itching. According to this concept, **cancer**, cardiovascular problems, joint problems, **dysentery**, **malaria**, **typhoid**, **gall stone**, **hemiplegia, tuberculosis**, **leprosy**, **polio**, **cholera** and all other diseases are due to psora which originated due to wrong thoughts.

"Homeopathy also says **psora** is the result of sinful thought while **sycosis** and **syphilis** are the result of sinful act. Without **psora, sycosis** and **syphilis** cannot be developed. These three are responsible for all chronic diseases."[159]

"Homeopathy also explains the cause of internal problems. This pathy says when skin diseases are treated by external application of ointment and lotion, it is very dangerous. External manifestations of **psora** in the form of skin disease if redirected internally are responsible for diseases of internal organs. When a person suffers from **psora**, **syphilis** and **sysosis** allopathic injection is given, it will internally direct the disease and make it incurable."[160]

Now, we can say that in Homeopathy treatment of skin diseases by external application of ointment and lotion is strictly contraindicated. Similarly injections also cannever be given. Do you accept thisconcept?

"A case of dysentery was described in Homeopathy and it was said that this was treated by arsenic, within 24 hours. A child of eight years old was suffering from fever, thirst and watery stool with foul smell 50 to 60 times in a day. This child was given arsenic of 30th potency. Within 24 hours patient became alright. The credit was given to Homeopathy."[161]

But what was the truth? "When a patient suffers from fever, diarrhoea, abdominal pain diagnosis may be shigellosis or bacillary dysentery. Other symptoms include nausea, vomiting, headache, myalgia, respiratory symptoms and in children, convulsions. This disease is an acute, self-limited infection of the intestinal tract of humans which is characterized by diarrhoea, fever and abdominal pain."[162]

There are various other causes of diarrhoea. Diagnosis of specific aetiological agent is done only by stool culture where specific bacteria and viral agent can be seen bymicroscope. Homeopathy does not accept external aetiology of disease. Bacteria and viruses are not accepted by Homeopathy therefore there is no question of specific diagnosis in Homeopathy.

"There are also other causes of **diarrhoea**. Most of the types are self-limiting."[163]

Not only Homeopathy but other useless pathies get unnecessary credit in these **diarrhoea** like diseases where diseases are actually self-limiting. In Homeopathy, drug is given in very dilute concentration and practically we can say that Homeopathic drugs contain no drug.

"Homeopathy also says that it is impossible to know about diseases. Homeopathy involves only in patients not in diseases. They take interest only in symptoms."[164]

"Homeopathy also says that body of a person cannot be diseased. Neither body nor any organ can get disease until and unless the psyche or thought process is not disturbed. Disease can spread only from mind to body. Body is actually an image of mind. If mind is pure no disease can exist in the body."[165]

It means that if a person has pure thought he cannot suffer from any disease. It also indicates that all diseases like **cancer**, **organ's enlargement, heart problems, thyroid disorders, diabetes, thyrotoxicosis, glomerulonephritis, peptic ulcer**, etc., are the result of disturbed psyche. According to Homeopathy, disturbed psyche is responsible for damage in various organs and causes disease.

"Disease first starts in mind or in psyche or in desire then it spreads in the body."[166] So when treatment is concerned treat psyche and desire of a patient. It is useless to treatdisease in Homeopathy, without treating psyche or thought. According to Homeopathy, diseases actually start from inside to outside of the body. According to Homeopathy, external factors like virus, bacteria, parasites, allergens, environmental agents cannot produce any disease.

Homeopathy always says that **tuberculosis**, **leprosy**, **typhoid**, **pneumonia** and other diseases are not caused by bacteria. These diseases are caused by wrong psyche and then spread from mind to body. This is the view of Homeopathy that bacteria and virus have no capacity to produce diseases, "first disease is produced then bacteria come and eat damaged portion of the organs."[167]

Today, this is totally a foolish concept that bacteria and virus are not responsible for any disease. Destruction of bacteria and virus by sterilization, antibiotics, chemotherapeutic agents and by vaccine improve health status of the world. Spread of diseases, epidemics and endemics are cured and checked by preventing spread of bacteria and viruses. Today, we know tropical diseases are caused by contaminated water. Epidemics occur after flood due to drinking of dirty water. Today, we also know that mosquitoes are responsible for**malaria** and **filaria**. If we accept Homeopathy then we shall have to agree with this concept that dirty water is not responsible for epidemics and mosquitoes do not cause **malaria**. Today, we have absolute evidence that mosquito causes **malaria** and bacteria causes diseases. This indicates that Homeopathy is illogical, unscientific and useless. Following examples explain pattern of treatment in Homeopathy.

"Here are four patients. One is suffering from bleeding in stomach, second is suffering from toothache with simple fever. Third patient is suffering from **diarrhoea** and fourth patient is suffering from **typhoid fever**. If all these patients have common symptoms like mental agony, thirst, desire for heat then treatment of all four patients will be the same like *arsenic*. If all the four patients are suffering from **cholera** with different mental symptoms, different desires, absence or presence of mental peace then treatment of **cholera** will be different for different patients."[168]

Typical concept of Homeopathy is that first of all mind is affected. Drug and disease both first influence the mind then body gets affected. According to Homeopathy, if a drugor disease has no effect on the mind it cannot influence the body.

Today, we know that there are hundreds of diseases and drugs which do not influence the mind but directly affect body. For example, **hypertension, diabetes, malaria, asthma, tumors, kidney disease, liver disease** are examples of disease where mind is not affected in the beginning.

Drugs acting on G.I.T., drugs acting on C.V.S., drugs acting on urinogenital system, drugs acting on respiratory system, drugs acting on skin, drugs acting on eye, all these drugs do not influence mind but directly influence organs and diseases are cured.

All tropical diseases are usually cured by antibiotics and chemotherapeutic agents without influencing mind. It proves that this concept of Homeopathy is also wrong. Homeopathy says— "External application of ointment or lotion in the skin disease should not be used. Injections are also not indicated in this therapy. These procedures suppress the disease. Body ejects faults of mind externally and makes mind pure. By wrong treatments external manifestations are suppressed and again redirected internally and damage internal organs. Then it has been wrongly understood that disease has been cured."[169]

23

Jealousy, lack of love, disturbed peace, selfishness, unfairness, unjustified attitude for others are the causative factors in the development of **psora. Psora** is the base of all diseases. Homeopathy divides all diseases into two groups—(1) New, (2) Old. If new diseases are treated wrongly, they convert into old or chronic diseases.

ARGUMENT

"Homeopathy divides all diseases into two groups—(1) New diseases, (2) Old diseases. New diseases are those diseases which may be resolved automatically. Either patient will die or patient will be cured automatically. If disease is strong then patient will die, but this disease will not remain in the body for prolonged period. Old diseases are those diseases which cannot be cured automatically. Such diseases remain in the body in various forms for prolonged duration."[170]

Homeopathy also says that if new diseases are treated wrongly, they convert into older chronic diseases. But what was the truth?

A large number of viral and bacterial diseases are cured automatically. If immunity is less or virulence of causative organism is great then there will be complications and disease will not be cured automatically. Due to these complications disease will remain in the body for prolonged duration. When these diseases are cured then Homeopathy says these diseases are new. When there are complications of disease Homeopathy says this is due to wrong treatment. This was the explanation given by Homeopathy. At that time when Homeopathy was originated, pathogenesis of disease was not known. When Homeopathy did not accept bacterial and viral aetiology of diseases then how could they have studied pathogenesis of disease. Homeopathy says complication of new disease always develops due to wrong treatment. But it is not true. Few patients of acute diseases have complications due to lack of immunity. "**Chickenpox** is a mild self-limiting disease. But this may be accompanied by severe complication particularly in immuno-suppressive patient and may also occur in normal children and adults. These include **haemorrhage**, **pneumonia**, **encephalitis**, acute **cerebella ataxia**."[171]

There are many other bacterial and viral diseases like**chickenpox**. Usually these infections are self-limiting. In few cases, there are complications and it was said wrongly that these were due to wrong treatment.

In those diseases where dehydration or blood loss is a problem, old allopathic treatment like shedding streams of blood and purgative complicate the diseases, *e.g.* in **cholera**.

But in those diseases where blood loss or dehydration is not a problem, external application of *mercurial ointment* or *cinchona bark* or *quinine*, can never convert diseases into chronic forms. Actually it was a wrong observation by supporters of Homeopathy. They understood complication of disease as complication ofmismanagement.

Hahnemann also said the same thing that "A human healing art, for the restoration to the normal state of those innumerable abnormal conditions often produced by the allopathic non-healing art, there is not and cannot be."[172]

One absurd concept of Homeopathy is **psora**. According to Homeopathy, all diseases are modification of **psora**. In the absence of **psora** disease is not possible. Jealousy, lack of love, disturbed peace, selfishness, unfairness, unjustified attitude towards others are the causative factors of development of**psora**. First mental stage of**psora** is developed. This mental itching of**psora** later appears on the surface in the form of physical itching. Presence of itching proves that there is**psora** in the body—

"In disease, state of mind reflects in the body."[173]

Hahnemann writes "The **psora**, the only real fundamental cause and producer of all the other numerous, I may say innumerable forms of diseases which come under the name of **nervous debility**, **hysteria**, **hypochondriasis, mania, melancholia, madness, epilepsy, convulsion** of all sorts, **scoliosis**, **hypnosis**, **caries**, **cancer**, **neoplasm**, **gout haemorrhoids, jaundice, cyanosis, dropsy, amenorrhoea, haemorrhage from the stomach, nose, lung, bladder, asthma, ulceration of lungs, of impotence**, and **barrenness**, of megrim, **deafness, cataract, amaurosis, urinary calculus, paralysis**, defect of senses and pain of thousands of kinds, etc."[174]

According to Homeopathy and Hahnemann, all the above written diseases are caused by only single agent **psora**. Today, we have knowledge regarding aetiology, pathology, diagnosis, investigation and treatment of diseases. We find different causative factors in different diseases. It is absolutely wrong to say that there is only one cause **psora** for all diseases.

Hahnemann did not mention character, morphology and measurement of **psora** and he also did not provide evidence of its existence. It is also said that this "extremely ancient infecting agent has gradually passed to some hundreds of generations through many millions of human organisms and has thus attained an incredible development, renders it in some measure, conceivable how it can now display such innumerable morbid forms in the great family of mankind."[175]

Again in this paragraph Hahnemann discarded external aetiological factors of diseases. According to Homeopathy, external factors alone can never create a disease. According to Homeopathy, a perfectly healthy man has no **psora** then administration of HIV virus or rabies virus in his body will not develop **AIDS** or **rabies** in him. Because in the absence of **psora** disease cannot be developed. Are supporters of Homeopathy ready to have administered HIV virus in their body? If they are not ready, then they are actually making fraudulent claims because they apply principles of Homeopathy on others but do not apply on themselves. According to Homeopathy they will not get **AIDS** by HIV virus.

24

Homeopathy opposes external application of lotion or ointment in skin diseases. This pathy says that skin diseases are not isolated problems, these are actually external manifestations of internal diseases. Local, surgical and other treatments for skin diseases are also not indicated in this therapy.

ARGUMENT

Another important fact regarding Homeopathy is that diseases which were self-limiting, Homeopaths claimed that they were treated by Homeopathy and those diseases which were not self-limiting Homeopaths said that diseases became chronic due to wrong treatment of Allopathy or no treatment. As said by Hahnemann:

"The true natural chronic diseases are those that arise from a chronic miasm, which when left to themselves and unchecked by the employment of those remedies that are specific for them, always go on increasing and growing worse... . These excepting those produced by medical malpractice, are the most numerous and greatest scourges of the human race."[176]

Homeopathy also defines what is the malpractice of Allopathy. "Homeopathy opposes external application of lotion or ointment in skin diseases. According to Homeopathy, skin diseases are external manifestations of **psora.** When these skin diseases are treated by external application of lotion and ointment, then these diseases are suppressed and directed internally and create severe internal diseases. According to this view skin diseases are not isolated problems, these are actually a part or external manifestation of internal diseases."[177] Conclusively we can say that those who are supporters of Homeopathy should never use external application of drugs in skin diseases. This means that either Homeopathy is true or skin specialist is true. Both can never be correct. Both are opposite to each other.

Similarly, Homeopathy also says that **psora, gonorrhea** and **syphilis** are suppressed by wrong treatment and this suppression creates so many complications in human body.

Hahnemann also writes—"It is not useful either in acute local diseases of recent origin or in local affections that have already existed a long time, to run in or apply external remedy, even though it be the specific and when used internally salutary by reason of its **Homeopathically**, even though it should be at the same time administered internally."[178]

"A product of **psora** which had hitherto remained latent in the interior, but has now burst forth is on the point of developing into a palpable chronic disease."[179]

This concept of Homeopathy says that skin diseases are a manifestation of **psora** and should not be suppressed.

"In chronic local maladies that are not obviously venereal the antipsoric internal treatment is more ever alone requisite."[180]

The above statement suggests that non-venereal local diseases like **boils, carbuncle, scabies, ring worm, local fungal infections, bed sores**, etc. are the external manifestations of **psora** and should not be treated locally. External treatment is prohibited in Homeopathy and only internal treatment is advised. It has also been said in Homeopathy:

"If the remedy perfectly Homeopathic to the disease had not yet been discovered at the time when the local symptoms were destroyed by a corrosive or desiccative external remedy or by the knife, then the cases become much more difficult on account of the too indefinite (uncharacteristic and inconstant) appearance of the remaining symptoms for what might have contributed most to determine the selection of the most suitable remedy and its internal employment until the disease should have been completely annihilated, namely the external principal symptoms have been removed from other observation."[181]

This paragraph says that all local symptoms are part of some general or systemic diseases and local problem should not be treated by external application of drug or by surgery. According to Homeopathy, presence of disease in body can be only diagnosed by external symptoms or visible external manifestations of disease. If external manifestations are removed by external application then Homeopath cannot decidewhether disease has been cured or remain in the body. By external application of drug, diseases redirect from external surface to interior of body and create complications. That's why Homeopathy opposes any type of external application of drug.

"The mere topical employment of medicines that are powerful for cure when given internally to the local symptoms of chronic miasmatic diseases is for the same reason quite inadmissible."[182]

Today, we know that above concept of Homeopathy is not true. Many diseases are treated only by local treatment. **Local abscess, cataract, conjunctivitis, glaucoma, deviated nasal septum, urethral structure, phimosis, localized carcinomatous growth,** are few examples where local treatment—surgical or medicinal is must. These diseases cannot be cured by internal treatment. Homeopathy says by the help of only external treatment local morbidity or local disease can never be treated. But at present we knowthat only localized surgical or medicinal treatment can cure these above ailments.

25

Warts are cured by internal application of Homeopathic drug. Localized extirpation of *carcinomatous* growth should not be done because that develops other internal diseases.

ARGUMENT

Hahnemann writes—"Persistence of local affections during its internal employment would have shown that the cure was not yet completed, but were it cured on its seat, this would be a convincing proof that the disease was completely eradicated of the desired recovery from the entire disease was fully accomplished, an estimable indispensable advantage to reach a perfect cure."[183]

Homeopathy says there is nothing like local disease or local affections. All local diseases are part of generalized internal diseases. Homeopathy also presumes that by only external application of drug, disease cannot be cured. For total eradication of disease drug should be given by oral route. Homeopathy says when external manifestations are removed after internal application of drug, it is a reliable indication of drug effect. Now, one example is being given here to explore this concept of Homeopathy.

"**Warts** are benign neoplasm of skin. **Warts** are found in approximately 7 to 20 per cent of the population. They occur mainly on skin areas unprotected by clothing except for the feet. **Warts** of several different clinical types are caused by the human papova viruses. **Warts** may persist and spread within the same person for several years or may recur in an individual several years after a total remission. Most studies indicate that one-third of **warts** are gone by six months and two-third of **warts** will resolve spontaneously within a two year period. **Condylomata acuminata** or **venereal warts** appear in the genital or anal area. Most **warts** will eventually spontaneously disappear without leaving any scars."[184]

In this example, **warts** disappear spontaneously within 6 to 24 months. In cases of **warts** if Homeopathic drug is given internally after presuming that **warts** are a part of general disease, then **warts** will be cured spontaneously and false reputation will be claimed by Homeopathy. In the treatment of **warts**, why are Homeopathy drugs are popular. The reality is not known by persons that **warts** are usually cured spontaneously. **Warts** are a strictly localized disease and resolve spontaneously. Homeopathy falsely claims that **warts** are cured by internal application of Homeopathic drug and makes wrong concept that **wart** is a part of general disease.

In this way, concept of Homeopathy and credit of Homeopathy depend on spontaneously curable diseases. As such Homeopathy plays no role in therapeutics.

According to Homeopathy there is nothing like localized disease. Homeopathy says localized diseases are part of generalized diseases. Hahnemann further explains, "It is evident that man's vital force, when encumbered with a chronic disease which it is unable to overcome by its own powers instinctively adopts the plan of developing a local malady on some external part... . It may thereby silence the internal disease which otherwise threatens to destroy the vital organs (and to deprive the patient of life) and that it may thereby, so to speak transfer the internal disease to the vicarious local affection... . The local affection however is never anything else than a part of it increased all in one direction by the organic vital force and transferred to a less dangerous (external part) of the body in order to allay the internal ailment."[185]

Hahnemann also made wrong generalizations of few diseases like **syphilis**. Hahnemann said, "The **chancre** enlarges as long as the internal **syphilis** remains uncured, old ulcers on legs get worse as long as the internal **psora** is uncured."[186]

In this way Hahnemann made generalization of knowledge based on only few diseases. In some cases local affections may be a part of general disease but it is not a universal truth. All local diseases are not part of general diseases. Homeopathy also opposes external application of drugs.

Hahnemann writes—"Physicians destroy the local symptoms by the topical application of external remedies, under the belief that he, thereby, cures the whole disease. Nature makes up for its loss by rousing the internal malady and the other symptoms that previously existed in a latent state side by side with the local affection that is to say though incorrectly that the local affection has been driven back into system or upon the nerves by the external remedies."[187]

Hahnemann also writes—"Burning away the **chancre** by caustics and destroying the **condylomata** on their seat by knife, the ligature or the actual cautery, this pernicious external mode of treatment is one of the most criminal procedures the medical world can be guilty of."[188] If Homeopathy is true then external treatment of localized affection should not be done, neither by knife nor by injection or drugs. If this concept of Homeopathy is true then skin specialist should not prescribe any local remedy, orthopaedicians should not use any local applications for non-traumatic localized disease. Localized **carcinomatous** growth should not be removed by surgery.

Why did Homeopathy oppose localized treatment?

Because Homeopathy concluded that localized treatment cannot cure localized diseases. It always aggravates the disease and deteriorate the condition of patients. Hahnemann also opposed local treatment by surgery.

Hahnemann writes—"I cannot advise for instance the local extirpation of the so called **cancer of the lips and face**... . The basic malady is, thereby, not diminished in slightest, the preserving vital force is, therefore, necessitated to transfer the field of operation of the great internal malady to some more important part (as it does in every case of metastasis) and the consequence is blindness, deafness, insanity, suffocative asthma... . The result is the same without previous cure of the inner miasm when **cancer of the face or breast** is removed by the knife alone and when encysted tumors areenucleated. Something worse ensues or at any rate death is hastened."[189]

Today, we know that the best and only treatment of carcinomatous growth is surgery.

The above conclusion of Hahnemann was wrong. Hahnemann did not know pathogenesis of spread of **cancer**. In many **cancers metastasis** occurs. **Cancer** usually spreads via lymph, blood into lung, liver, brain, bone and other parts of body. If **carcinomatous** growth is removed early, it will not spread and if there is delay in removal ofgrowth it will spread in the body. Hahnemann thought wrongly that it was the surgical removal of **cancer** which was responsible for spread of **cancer** in body and surgical removal was not the real treatment because even after surgical treatment patient suffered by metastatic growth. Due to lack of knowledge Hahnemann got wrong impressions and presented a wrong pathy to the world.

Hahnemann also concluded wrongly that external removal of carcinomatous growth produces other internal diseases. Actually what happens if there is carcinomatous growth of advanced stage, there will be **metastasis**. Even after removal of carcinomatous growth by surgery these **metastasis** which is already present in different parts of body produce different signs and symptoms according to organ involved.

The pattern of metastatic spread is different in different **cancers**. If a part of **cancer** reaches in the brain, neurological signs and symptoms will be the result. If metastatic growth reaches the lung, respiratory problems will be the result. In this way different types of signs and symptoms will be produced according to the organ involved. Hahnemann said by mistake that these different types of signs and symptoms are the result of different types of internal diseases produced due to the removal of carcinomatous growth by surgery. Here Hahnemann was absolutely wrong for delivering a wrong message to the world.

26

Rapid increase of the psychiatric symptoms is related to improvement in corporal symptoms. Hahnemann prescribed *aconite*, *belladonna*, *hyoscyamus, mercury* in highly potentized minute Homeopathic doses.

ARGUMENT

Hahnemann writes regarding allopathic treatment of psychiatric patient that, "In Allopathy psychiatric patients are managed by harsh and cruel behaviors. Physical tortures are given to psychiatric patients and they are behaved like criminals."[190]

Hahnemann criticized rightly the treatment of old Allopathy. "The earliest treatment of mental disorder was exorcism which included prayer, incantation, noise making, flogging, starving and other more severe measures. There were also patients who were beheaded or strangled before being burned, burned alive and some were mutilated before being burned."[191]

But today, these methods are not used in treatment of psychiatric patients. In modern medical science which is also called modern Allopathy for the treatment ofpsychiatric patients drugs, psychotherapy and sociotherapy are used. These methods are human methods. Now a large percentage of psychiatric patients can be cured completely and they are able to live normal life.

Now again we can say Hahnemann opposed old Allopathy. At the time of Hahnemann, there was no existence of modern developed medical science. So this statement that Hahnemann opposed modern medical science is absolutely wrong.

Hahnemann writes "Almost all the so-called mental and emotiona diseases are nothing more than corporeal diseases in which the symptoms of derangement of the mind and disposition peculiar to each of them is increased whilst the corporeal symptoms decline. The cases are not rare in which a so-called corporeal that threatens to be fatal a suppuration of lung or the deterioration of some other important viscous or some other disease of acute character... becomes transformed into insanity, into a kind or **melancholia** or into **mania** by a rapid increase of the psychiatric symptoms that were previously present where upon the corporeal symptoms lose all their danger, these later improve almost to perfect health.... ."[192]

These observations of Hahnemann were wrong. It does not mean that Hahnemann was not intelligent. He was definitely very intelligent but due to lack of necessary information and poor available knowledge, he was not able to reach on right conclusion. At present we know that "All mental and emotional diseases are not the result of corporeal diseases. Some psychiatric symptoms are the result of organic diseases. One example is **delirium**. **Delirium** is characterized by clouding of consciousness, perceptual disturbance, incoherent speech, disorientation and memory impairment, variability of clinical features from time to time and most importantly a specific organic factor or factors thought to be the cause of the disturbance.

Excess mortality is due to the nature of disease that causes **delirium**. Progression to irreversible organic brain syndromes is sometimes observed, especially in those cases in which the aetiology cannot be treated effectively."[193]

When psychiatric symptoms increase, intensity of corporeal disease does not decline in cases of **delirium**. If organic diseases, responsible for **delirium** are not treated effectively then chances of death become more. This conclusion is against the "*Organon of Medicine*" which says that when psychiatric symptoms increase, corporeal symptoms loss all their danger. For the treatment of **delirium** Hahnemann prescribed "*aconite*, *belladonna, hyoscyamus*, *mercury*, *stramonium* in highly potentized, minute Homeopathic doses."[194]

These drugs prescribed for the treatment of **delirium** when given in high doses produces delirium with other toxic signs and symptoms.

Aconite produces "sometimes **delirium** or convulsion, insensibility and coma."[195]

By **stramonium,** hypocrite and belladonna in high doses "patient becomes restless, markedly excited and delirious. Delirium is of a particular character. He is silent or mutters indistinct inaudible words but usually he is noisy, tries to run away from his bed, tries to pull imaginary threads from the tips of his fingers and is subject to dreadful hallucinations of sight and hearing."[196]

During mercury poisoning "**Neuropsychiatric** symptoms also occur."[197]

All these drugs produce **delirium** and other psychiatric symptoms when given **in toxic** doses but these drugs cannot cure **delirium**. When drugs are given in Homeopathic doses in high dilutions, these drugs don't have any effect on human body. They are neither therapeutic nor toxic. Regarding Homeopathic doses, we can say that they are not drugs at all.

Homeopathic dose means no drug but how Hahnemann got some positive results by these drugs in **delirium**?

There are various causes of **delirium**. Bacterial, viral infections and toxic dose of various drugs also cause **delirium**. Many infections like typhoid and viral infections are self-limiting. Toxic substance, responsible for **delirium** gradually metabolise in the body and **delirium** subsides spontaneously if there is no irreversible damage in the brain. Systemic infections like fever also cause delirium. As infections and fever are cured, **delirium** also gets cured. In this way delirium may be resolved automatically without any treatment. In such conditions Homeopathy gets **pseudo-reputation** as a treating agent.

Facts about **delirium** should be known to all.

"It is not too unusual for **delirium** to come and go without a specific cause being identified."[198] Actually what happens? If a patient is cured by Homeopathy then it is said it is Homeopathic drugs which are responsible for cure, irrespective of spontaneous cure of disease. If disease is not cured by Homeopathic drug then it is said that allopathic drug or some other treatments have spoiled case and that's why Homeopathic drug could not cure the patient.

Actually, "Acute brain disorders are caused by diffused impairment of brain function. Such impairment may result from a variety of conditions including high fevers, nutritional deficiency and drug intoxication. Symptoms range from mild mood changes to acute delirium. The prognosis in acute brain disorder is good, such conditions usually clear up over a short period of time."[199]

27

According to Homeopathy, **dilution** and **trituration** increase the potency of a drug. The material part of the medicine is lessened with each degree of *dynamization* 50,000 times and yet incredibly increased in power. The 30th *thus progressively prepared would* give a fraction almost impossible to be expressed in number but highly potent in power.

ARGUMENT

Now I am describing the method of preparing Homeopathic medicine. It is said that by this method crude medicinal substances develop their curative power to the utmost which is as follows: "One grain of the powdered drug is triturated with 100 grains of sugar of milk. The powder thus prepared is put in a vial well corked, protected from direct sunlight to which designation of the first product marked $\overline{100}$ is given. Now one grain of the powdered 100 is mixed and triturated with 100 grains of powdered sugar of milk and then labelled $\overline{10000}$. Now again one grain of this powder is mixed and triturated with 100 grains of powdered sugar of milk and this is labelled as $\overline{1000000}$. One grain of this powder contains 1/1000000 of the original substance. One grain of this powder is dissolved in 500 drops of a mixture of one part of alcohol and four parts of distilled water of which one drop is put in a vial. To this are added 100 drops of pure alcohol and 100 strong or successions are given. This is the medicine of first degree **dynamization.** Small sugar globules are then moistened with this fluid and quickly spread on blotting paper to dry and kept in a vial with the sign of degree of potency.

To prepare drug of 2 degree of potency take one sugar globule of first degree and dissolve in another vial with one drop of water, then add 100 drops of good alcohol and **dynamize** with this medicinal fluid. Sugar globules are again moistened and dried quickly on blotting paper and give the sign of II potency.

In this way, drug upto 30th potency should be made."[200] Regarding such dilution, Hahnemann writes:

"I have found after many laborious experiments and counter experiments that the material part of the medicine is lessened with each degree of dynamization 50000 times and yet incredibly increased in power. The 30th thus progressively prepared would give a fraction almost impossible to be expressed in numbers."[201]

Homeopathic drugs contain such dilutions that practically these dilutions contain no drug at all. Homeopathic drugs actually contain no drug. Homeopathic drugs have no curative and therapeutic power. In other words, these drugs have no effect on the body. Hahnemann says by **succussions** medicinal power of a drug is increased. By knowledge of physics we know by succussions only mechanical energy is produced which is responsible for slight increase in temperature and nothing else.

"In Homeopathy, dilutions are based on a 1:10 ratio represented by the Roman numeral X or D, and centesimal based on a 1:100 ratio by the Roman letter C. Hence a 1X Homeopathic dosage is 10 fold dilution, 2X is a 100 fold dilution, 3X is a 1000 fold dilution, etc. The 1C represents a 100 fold dilution, 2C is a 10,000 fold dilution and 3C is a 1,000,000 fold dilution, etc. Most Homeopathic remedies range from 6X (one part in a million) to 30X (one part in 10^{30})."[202]

In such dilutions there is actually no drug molecule. When there is no drug molecule, how can we expect that it can have any effect on the body. "According to the laws of chemistry, there is a point at which a substance can be diluted so that no more remains. The limit is referred to as Avogadro's number, which closely corresponds to the Homeopathic dosage of 24X (one part in 10^{-24}). Even Hahnemann recognized that in all likelihood, extreme dilutions would not contain a single molecule of the original material."[203]

28

Homeopathy opposes treatment of fever. **Tuberculosis** and similar diseases are developed when fever is treated. This pathy says only presence of symptoms indicates the disease. If investigations indicate that there are no symptoms, Homeopathy would not accept the disease. During treatment, first mind gets cured only then body is cured. Homeopaths criticized injections and vaccinations. They say these procedures are very dangerous.

ARGUMENT

"Homeopathy opposes treatment of fever. By treatment of fever Homeopathy says, size of liver and spleen is increased. **Tuberculosis** and other similar diseases are developed when fever is treated.'[204] Today we know temperature above 102°F is dangerous to the body. **Hyperpyrexia** is also responsible for death, but it is Homeopathy which says that fever should not be **treated** and diseases like tuberculosis originated due to the treatment of fever. This is Homeopathy. "Homeopathy says if external symptoms of disease are improved but patient is not feeling well, and he is not calm and quite, then we cannot say that patient is improving."[205] In this case treatment is not accurate. "This pathy says that external symptoms (like fever, pain, frequency of stool, cough, dyspnoea) are increased in severity and patient feels better then it indicates patient is improving."[206] The mechanism of above action is explained as follows: first drug acts inside and patient feels better, then drug acts outside. Action of drug starts from inside to outside, that's why first patient feels good, then symptoms are removed. Persons having little knowledge of medical science knows well that first external symptoms are improved then only patient feels better. For example if a patient is suffering from fever of 105°F, first we have to reduce his temperature then only will the patient feel better. It is not possible that first patient will feel better then only temperature will be reduced. Similar statement is true if patient is suffering with severe pain. Without removing pain patient cannot feel good.

Improvement in external symptoms like pain, fever, swelling are definite signs of cure but Homeopathy denies this. How can patient improve or feel well when he is suffering from severe pain or high grade temperature or with deteriorating symptomatology?

Homeopaths criticized vaccination and injections. "According to these experts, vaccination and injections create various complications and they say these procedures are very dangerous."[207]

But we know that injections of various medicines are life-saving in emergencies. Besides this many drugs are administered only by injections. Vaccinations are highly beneficial in preventing many infectious diseases. In vaccinations, vaccines are administered which prevent the development of disease. *Vaccine* is an *immunobiological* substance designed to produce specific protection against a given disease. It stimulates the production of protective antibody of other immune mechanism. **In Smallpox, rabies, cholera, diphtheria, tuberculosis, pertusis, tetanus, influenza, yellow fever, mumps, polio, measles, rubella, hepatitis-B** vaccines are used in the prevention of respective diseases. In May 1974, the W.H.O. officially launched a global immunization program as expanded program on immunization to protect all children of the world against six vaccine preventable diseases namely **diphtheria, whooping cough, tetanus, polio, tuberculosis** and **measles** by the year 2000. "One effective way to control the spread of infection is to strengthen the host's defense mechanism. Under certain circumstances this may be accomplished by active immunization which is one of the most powerful and cost effective weapon of modern medicines. There are some infectious diseases whose control is solely based on active immunization *e.g.* **Polio, tetanus, diphtheria, measles**. Immunization is a mass means of protecting the greatest number of people."[208]

Today if an expert or a pathy opposes vaccinations and says that vaccination and immunization are harmful then we can say that these persons are fools and these pathies are useless.

29

If two dissimilar diseases meeting together in the human being are of equal strength or if the older one be the stronger, the new disease will be repelled by the old one from the body and not allowed to affect it or, strong disease suppresses another weak disease. When stronger disease is cured, weaker disease reappears.

ARGUMENT

Here again detailed analysis of argument no. 10 is being given because this topic is very important when analysis of Homeopathy is concerned.

Hahnemann made some observations and on the basis of these observations Hahnemann developed Homeopathy. At the time of Hahnemann medical science was not developed. **Aetiology**, pathogenesis, specific diagnosis, investigations, were not well known. Hahnemann himself did not believe in diagnosis, investigations, pathogenesis and exogenous **aetiological** agents. Hahnemann made this wrong conclusion.

"If two dissimilar diseases meeting together in the human being be of equal strength or still more if the older one be the stronger, the new disease will be repelled by the old one from the body and not allowed to affect it."[209]

The above wrong conclusion of Hahnemann was also based on the "following observations."[210]

1. A patient suffering from severe chronic disease will not be infected by a moderate autumnal **dysentery** or other epidemic disease.
2. Those suffering from **pulmonary tuberculosis** are not liable to be attacked by epidemic fever of not very violent character.
3. **Pulmonary phthisis** remained stationary when the patient was attacked by a violent **typhus**.
4. In an epidemic, **measles** attacked many individuals on the fourth and fifth days after the inoculation of **smallpox** and prevented the development of **smallpox**.
5. The **mumps** immediately disappear when the **cowpox** inoculation had taken effect.
6. **Smallpox** coming on after vaccination at once remove and entirely the **cowpox** Homeopathically.
7. The fever accompanying **cowpox** cured Homeopathically intermittent fever in two individuals.
8. In some, two fevers cannot coexist in the same body.
9. In an epidemic where **measles** and **whooping cough** prevailed, many children who took **measles** remained free from **whooping cough** etc.

Hahnemann also said that many diseases have been Homeopathically cured by other diseases presenting similar symptoms.

Today we can say:

By the symptoms only a disease cannot be diagnosed with confirmation. For infective diseases, viral and bacterial isolation and its confirmation microscopically or by serologically test is must. Hahnemann may have made this mistake and concluded wrong interpretations after wrong diagnosis. And by observing one or two or few cases nothing can be concluded. Immunity plays a very important rolein development of a disease. Hahnemann did not know about immunity and antigen antibody reaction that's why he did not understand the mechanism of above observations.

In the development of a disease, resistance of the host is very important. Resistance means ability to localize and destroy micro-organism. This capacity is dependent upon the presence of specific antibody that synthesizes in response to specific antigenic stimulus. Variations in host resistance are result of host's ability to form antibody. Malnutrition (especially protein deficiency), toxic depression due to bacterial toxins, hormonal imbalance can greatly depress synthesis of antibody. Anything that reduces number of leucocytes also reduces resistance.

Very young and very old persons are much more susceptible to bacterial disease. New-born infant has little capacity for producing antibody until he is several months of age. "Presence of other disease may greatly reduce resistance to bacterial infection. **Diabetic** patients are predisposed to infections of skin and urinogenital tract. **Influenza**, **measles** and other viral infections of lung markedly predispose to secondary bacterial infection. **Silicosis** is associated with a striking increase in susceptibility to **tuberculosis**. **Malnutrition**, exhaustion, shock, exposure to cold, chronic alcoholism, psychic disturbances, etc. may also seriously interfere with the individual's resistance to bacterial disease."[211]

"Prior contact with an organism or its product whether by active infection or by artificial immunization increases resistance to some infections such as **measles**, **diphtheria** and **pertusis** by stimulating antibody production."[212]

We also know today that immunity creates resistant state but some forms of immune reaction rather than providing exemption or safety can produce severe and occasionally fatal results, it is known as hypersensitivity reaction. It is actually inappropriate response to an antigenic stimulus which may be a self molecule or a drug or microbial product. Microbial product means product from bacteria, virus or protozoa or other micro-organism. "Examples are**salmonella infection**, **tubercular infection**, **leprosy**, **streptococcal infection**. Clinical manifestations depend upon where the antigen antibody complexes form or lodge. Skin, joints, kidney and heart are main site. In hypersensitivity reaction eczema, skin rashes, pyrexia, **arthralgia** may be developed. These events occur in drug ingestion, bacterial and viral infection".[213]

"Immunity also plays a protective role in **polio** and a number of other viral infections. Immunity to many viral infection is life-long.'[214]

"It is also known that infections with **influenza**, **rubella**, **measles** and other viruses predispose to bacterial and other infections."[215]

"Susceptibility to infection is generally greater in the title young ones and olds because of a weaker immune response. However, the **immunopathology** tends to be less severe."[216]

"Natural infection from a virus is an extremely effective means of giving life-long immunity from the disease. In most cases where there is one virus type, it means that second attacks are extremely rare" [217] "because of the intimate relationship of viruses to the metabolism of their host cells, immunity may be raised or lowered by nutritional changes, endocrinal disturbances, heat, cold, shock, radiation and other factors that stimulate or inhibit the activity of intracellular enzymes."[218]

This fact of antigen-antibody reaction in viral and bacterial infection was missed by Hahnemann and this is also responsible in the development of Homeopathy.

If immunity is strong then some diseases may be totally **asymptomatic** *e.g.* "**Rubella** is a mild self limiting viral disease and there is evidence that the disease may be entirely **asymptomatic** and detectable only by **leucopenia** and lymph node enlargement."[219] This shows that disease may exist in the body without anysymptoms. In such conditions Hahnemann may have thought it was the absence of disease and made wrong conclusions but in fact there was disease.

Viral infections usually have characteristically specific skin lesions. In some viral infections skin lesions are the only manifestations *e.g.* in **chickenpox**.

"In the great majority of cases the **cutaneous** eruption is the only lesion seen"[220] and in **measles** "there is an **erythematous cutaneous** eruptions of a characteristic appearance.'[221] "**Herpes zoster**, commonly known as **shingles** is characterized by the formation of an**erythematous** and vesicular eruption along thecourse of sensory nerves."[222] Similarly, **smallpox** and **chickenpox** have characteristic skin lesions. It is also known that "antigen-antibody reactions are important in causing **cutaneous** eruption *e.g.* note the absence of rashes in **measles** when antibodies do not form"[223] That's why we can tell when antigen—antibody reaction is weak then skin manifestations will be less and organs where antigen antibody complex causes damage will also be less. In such conditions diagnosis of disease is difficult due to the absence of characteristically-specific skin lesions and less morbidity due to diminished antigen antibody reaction or less hypersensitivity reaction.

Hahnemann did not know about complexity. Definitely he made a mistake regarding presence and absence of disease and made a wrong conclusion for example Hahnemann observed that two similar diseases cannot exist together. This observation was based on the absence of one disease. If **cutaneous** lesions are absent and morbidity is less then one may think of absence of disease because at the time of Hahnemann these were the only criteria for the presence or absence of disease in the body but absent **cutaneous** lesions and diminished morbidity gave the wrong impression that disease was absent. Definitely this was the mistake made by Hahnemann and he thought wrongly that one disease cures similar disease but in fact one disease diminishes immunity which makes antigen-antibody reaction less strong. This gives the false impression that disease is absent.

This explanation can be easily proved with the help of **AIDS** patients and patients of **tuberculosis**.

"Tuberculin is a test material or antigen derived from tubercular bacteria when injected intradermally in the forearm, a positive reaction consistins of erythema and induration is accepted as evidence of past or present infection by mycobacterium **tuberculosis**. It is actually an antigen antibody reaction. If cellular immunity is poor then by negative tuberculin test **tuberculosis** cannot be excluded. The dermal hypersensitivity to tuberculin can also be lost in variousstates of immune suppression *e.g.* **malignancy, Hodgkin's disease**."[224]

AIDS, the Acquired Immuno Deficiency Syndrome, is a fatal illness caused by a retrovirus known as the human **immuno** deficiency virus which destroys the body's immune system. Then patient becomes vulnerable to various dangerous infections, neurological disorders and malignancies.

A **HIV** infected patient (that is human **immuno** deficiency virus infection or **HIV** infection which causes AIDS) "with tuberculosis have a higher frequency of false negative tuberculin skin test. HIV positive people with **pulmonary tuberculosis** may have a higher frequency of negative sputum smears. In people with HIV who do not have a fully functioning immune system, there is less tissue destruction and hence less lung cavitations. Cavities usually develop because of the immune response to the tubercular bacilli."[225]

Decreased immunity is responsible for less damage in only those organs where antigen antibody complex is responsible for destruction of tissue. It does not mean that there is no symptoms or there is no disease or disease will remain symptom-less. Micro-organisms also produce detrimental effect in body byvarious other methods like toxins, interference in cellular metabolism, septicemia,etc. Decreased immunity by first infection interfered in skin manifestations and in some cases it may decrease symptomatology which confused Hahnemann who then made wrong interpretation.

I am again explaining one example of how Hahnemann made a wrong conclusion. Due to lack of knowledge Hahnemann writes— "**Small pox** coming on after vaccination as its great similarity at once remove entirely the **cowpox** homeopathically and does not permit it to come to maturity but on the other hand, **cowpox** when reaches near maturity on account of its great similarity homeopathically diminish very much the supervening **smallpox** and make it much milder."[226]

Hahnemann concluded that **cowpox** and **smallpox** both prevent development of each other. Both diseases have similar **symptomatology**. So Hahnemann said that one disease homeopathically cured another disease. Hahnemann gave emphasis on similar **symptomatology**, but what was the truth?

It was not the similarity in **symptomatology** of **cowpox** and **smallpox** which cured each other but it was the immunological and serological similarity of both types of viruses. **Smallpox** is caused by **variola** virus. **Cowpox** is also a viral disease. By knowledge of pathology we know "**Cowpox** virus resembles that of **smallpox** morphologically and **immunologically** and the histological changes in the skin at the site of vaccination are essentially identical with those of **smallpox**."[227]

Cowpox virus and **smallpox** virus both are similar **immunologically**. This means both have similar antigenic structures. They make common antibodies. Antibodies developed after **cowpox** inoculation prevents development of **smallpox** and vice versa. It is not the similarity in **symptomatology** but similarity in **(immunological)** antigenic structure which prevent other disease by formation of common antibodies. **Cowpox** virus develops antibodies which also kill **smallpox** virus and **smallpox** viruses develop antibodies which also kill **cowpox** viruses. This is the actual mechanism.

Empirical observation of therapeutic benefits in few cases and actual therapeutical benefits both are two different aspects, as cleared by the following paragraph:

"In the past **vaccinia** virus had also been occasionally used for the treatment of disease such as recurrent **herpes**, **simplex infection** or **warts**. There is no evidence of therapeutic efficacy in these situations and the use of the virus for these purposes is strictly contraindicated.'[228]

Hahnemann says that two dissimilar diseases cannot exist in the body together and he himself mentioned such examples which are against the homeopathic concept.

"**Smallpox** and **measles**, both these dissimilar diseases were present at the same time. There was also a case where **cowpox** runs its regular course along with **measles** and along with purpura."[229]

There are many examples of dissimilar diseases which exist together. Diabetic patients also suffer from **malaria**, **hypertension**, **cardiac problems** and other diseases.

Hypertensive patient also get infective disease or other non-tropical diseases like **cancer**, **renal** and **cardiac diseases**.

According to Homeopathy, if a person is suffering from a chronic disease then during this period he cannot suffer from any other disease having dissimilar **symptomatology**. What homeopathy says is that if a person is suffering from **diabetes** or **hypertension** or **cancer** he cannot suffer from any other disease like **malaria**, **typhoid**, **dysentery**.

Do you agree with this concept? Can you accept such irrational comments?

By the knowledge of *interferon* we can analyze various observations of Hahnemann. Hahnemann did not know about*interferon* that's why he made wrong conclusions.

"*Interferons* are species specific cellular glycoprotein, produced naturally by virus infected cells and have antiviral protective action. They are capable of interfering with a wide variety of DNA and RNA viruses. They can, therefore, be considered as potent broad spectrum antiviral compound with a high therapeutic ratio."[230]

"Certain agents like the live attenuated measles virus, bacterial **endotoxins,** other microbial extracts, polysaccharides can stimulate the production of endogenous *interferon.*"[231]

"The enhanced production of the antiviral proteins called *interferons* is one of the body's earliest responses to a viral infection. It is thought that the *interferons* help contain viral infections until the immune system can be fully activated. All cells appear to have the capacity to produce these substances after exposure to appropriate stimulus, virus a protozoan parasite, lipo polysaccharides or an antibiotic such as kanamycin is all that is needed to increase a cell's rate of interferon synthesis. It is known that *interferon* can prevent viruses from reproducing. The *interferons* in addition to being used to treat viral infections are being extensively investigated for use in **AIDS** and **Cancer therapy**."[232]

"*Interferons* may ameliorate viral infections by exerting direct antiviral effect and/or by modifying the immune response to infection."[233] By the above studies it is clear that viral infection, **protozoal** infection create *interferon* in the host. That *interferon* prevents or suspends next consequent viral infection by antiviral action.

This fact was not known to Hahnemann that one infection prevents next infection by producing *interferon*. When Hahnemann observed in viral diseases that one infection prevents second infection of similar **symptomatology** he made the wrong law that one disease is cured by disease of similar **symptomatology**. He applied this observation in all diseases which was wrong.

Protozoal infection also develops *interferon* which can prevent further viral infection. *Interferon* is also *synthesized* by various other stimulatory agents. This is sufficient to say that conclusion of Hahnemann was not accurate because one viral infection may prevent development of another viral or bacterial infection irrespective of similarity or dissimilarity in **symptomatology**.

30

In tuberculosis, killing of *mycobacteria* will kill the patient. If we could succeed today in putting a fluid into the anatomy that would destroy the bacteria that consumptive would die soon.

ARGUMENT

James Kent is another name which is highly respected in the field of Homeopathy. Lectures on homeopathic philosophy by James Kent are being popular. Kent said in his lectures—

"Tubercles come first and the bacillus is secondary. It has never been found prior to the tubercle, but it follows that. Bacilli are not the cause of disease, they never come until after the disease.... Hahnemann did not adopt any such theory of bacteriology... . If we could succeed today in putting a fluid into the anatomy that would destroy the bacteria that consumptive would die soon."[234] Today, we know with certainty that "**Tuberculosis** is a specific infective disease caused by a bacteria mycobacterium tuberculosis. **Tuberculosis** chemotherapy has been one of the most significant advances during this century. With the evolution of controlled trials, the chemotherapy of **tuberculosis** is now more rationally based than in the treatment of other infectious diseases. The objective of chemotherapy treatment is cure that is the elimination of both the fast and slowly multiplying bacilli from the patient's body."[235]

Kent says that killing of mycobacterium **tuberculosis** will kill the patient. It means antibiotic or chemotherapeutic drugs which kill the bacteria will not cure the disease but will be responsible for death of patients. Death will be increased by chemotherapeutic agents. Today, we know that this above concept of Kent and Hahnemann is absolutely wrong. Now a days—"Antituberculosis chemotherapy has reduced the mortality of **miliary tuberculosis** from 100 per cent to less than 5 per cent. Prognosis is excellent in primary **pulmonary tuberculosis** and its complications. Now fatal outcome is extremely uncommon, even if the disease has reached an advanced stage.'[236] Homeopathy rejects bacterial cause of disease but chemotherapeutic agents that kill bacteria are effective against diseases. Antibiotics are substances that kill micro-organisms and "approximately 30 per cent of all hospitalized patients receive one or more courses of therapy with antibiotics and millions of potentially fatal infections have been cured."[237]

Still persons of medical science have faith in Homeopathy, this indicates that they do not understand the basic principles of therapeutics. They get the medical degree but they do not get medical knowledge. Actually there should not be such divisions in therapeutic systems like Allopathy, Ayurveda, Homeopathy, Yoga therapy, etc. We should give this message to the society that whatever is correct and proven by experimental studies is modern medical science. And whatever is empirical, not proven by experimental studies and is incorrect is not modern medical science. Such facts should be known to all medical persons and it should be taught to medical students.

The basics of Homeopathy are wrong. Then derivations based on these basics will be definitely wrong. When we are sure that basic principles of Homeopathy are wrong then not a single disease can be cured by homeopathic method of treatment. If some diseases are benefited by homeopathic drug then it is sure that there is either spontaneous recovery of the disease or placebo reaction.

Similarly we can explain various observations made by Hahnemann and we can say with certainty that the conclusion drawn by Hahnemann was wrong.

Support of Ayurveda, Homeopathy and other non-scientific methods of treatment is actually a crime. Because this support is responsible for so many deaths of uneducated citizens especially villagers. Poor people and people from villages take Ayurveda and Homeopathy and suffer a lot. Many people die or become disabled. Preventable disease are spreading dangerously in India. I know many people who were taking Ayurvedic or Homeopathic treatment for **tuberculosis** and ultimately these people died. Many people first take medical treatment for one or two months then start Homeopathy or Ayurveda. **Tuberculosis** treatment should be taken 6 to 12 months continuously for complete treatment. The**tuberculosis** of these patients become resistant and then it is impossible to treat. Such foolishness is responsible for spreading many diseases like **malaria** and **tuberculosis**.

The emergence of drug resistant strains of micro-organisms or parasites is promoted by treatments that do not result in cure."[238]

31

Kent said persons suffering from **diabetes**, **tuberculosis** and **Bright's disease** cannot suffer from another dissimilar mild infections like **dysentery**.

ARGUMENT

"Kent has also said in his lectures that dissimilar disease can suspend another disease. He also said if a person has some form of mild chronic disease, a severe attack of dysentery will cause that disease to disappear temporarily and the new disease will take hold and run its course and when it subsides the old symptoms will come back again."[239]

According to his opinion, if the previous disease is strong then subsequent disease if dissimilar cannot suppress previous disease. Kent has mentioned some examples which were the basis of the above conclusions. "A number of persons who**are anything but strong really invalids**, one in consumption, another in the last stages of **Bright's disease**, another with **diabetes**. We called them all together and find that none of them have had **dysentery** or **smallpox** or whatever disease was epidemic"[240]

Kent said in his lecture that persons suffering from **diabetes**, **tuberculosis**, **Bright's disease** cannot suffer from another dissimilar mild infections like **dysentery** and **smallpox**.

These observations are very important because Homeopathy is based on these observations. If we can prove that these observations are wrong then undoubtedly we can say that Homeopathy is also wrong. Kent observed that patients of **diabetes**, **tuberculosis** and **Bright's disease** cannot suffer from any other infection like **dysentery** or **small-pox**. But what are the facts?

"**Diabetic** patients also suffer from **diarrhoea**."[241] Other diseases having dissimilar **symptomatology** also exist with **diabetes** and it is against the rule of Homeopathy that diseases of dissimilar **symptomatology** cannot exist together in a patient. **Malignant external otitis, rhinocerebral mycormycosis** which is characterized by periorbitaland perinasal swelling, pain, bloody nasal discharge and increased lacrimation, also exist with diabetes. "Diabetes is characterized by thirst, **polydipsia**, **polyuria**, **nocturia**, tiredness, loss of weight, white marks on clothing, impotence, **pruritis** vulvae and **parasthesiae** or pain in limbs."[242] **Emphysematous cholecystitis** is a variant of gall bladder disease that tends to affect diabetic men. "Infestations of the skin with **Candida** and **dermatophytes** are common and bacterial infections of variety of types that also occur."[243] Homeopathy says two similar diseases cannot exist in the body because one disease cures another disease of similar **symptomatology.**

Homeopathy also says that two diseases of dissimilar **symptomatology** cannot exist together in the body because one disease will suspend another disease.

Tuberculosis and **HIV** have different **symptomatology** but both diseases may remain in single patient together. We observed "World-wide, the number of people infected with both **HIV** and **tuberculosis** is rising. To make the global situation worse **tuberculosis** has formed a lethal partnership with **HIV**." [244]

This observation is against the Kent's view that **tuberculosis** patient cannot suffer from other disease.

HIV infection is associated with various diseases of similar and dissimilar symptomatology. "70 per cent of **HIV** infected people experience fever, rash and sore throat, a few weeks after initial infection of **HIV**. **Tuberculosis, kaposi sarcoma, inflammation of retina in cytomegalovirus retinitis,** dry non-productive cough, weight loss, fever in **pneumocystis-carinii**, **pneumonia**, mild **hemiplegla** and other neurological signs and symptoms in **toxoplasma encephalitis**; fever, headache, vomiting, neck stiffness in **cryptococcal meningitis**, pain and burning sensation, skin blisters in **herpes zoster** and other skin infections are usually associated with **HIV** infection."[245]

What conclusion can be drawn by analyzing above paragraph? Disease of similar and dissimilar symptomatology can exist together. If it is true then the concept of Homeopathy is wrong.

Subclinical infections and latent infections confused Hahnemann and Kent. In subclinical cases "disease agent may multiply in the host but does not manifest itself by signs and symptoms. Persons who are thus sick unknown to themselves and others barring a few *e.g.* measles, subclinical infection occurs in most infectious diseases. In some diseases *e.g.* **rubella, mumps, polio, hepatitis A** and **B, Japanese encephalitis, influenza**, **diphtheria**, a great deal of subclinical infections occur frequently during a person's lifetime, they are responsible for the immunity."[246]

"In latent infection the host does not shed the infectious agent which lies dormant within the host without symptoms *e.g.* latent infection occurs in **herpes simplex**, infections due to slow viruses."[247]

Hahnemann and Kent gave importance to symptoms only. They did not understand the presence of microbe inside the body. Whenever immunity weakens, subclinical infections manifest as signs and symptoms. If there are no symptoms then they say that there is no disease.

For example, viral infection produces *interferon*—an antiviral substance which also prevents further viral infection. If *interferon* is not in sufficient amount, then there may be chances that second subsequent infection may remain in subclinical formwithout producing signs and symptoms. Hahnemann may have observed in this case that previous disease prevented development of second disease. But in fact second disease remained in subclinical form.

Hahnemann and Kent did not know about subclinical and latent infection which were also responsible for their wrong conclusions.

Subclinical infection, can be detected only by laboratory tests*e.g.* antibody response, recovery of the organisms, skin sensitivity and biochemical tests.

For analytical study, knowledge of subclinical infection and latent infection is important. Similarly concept of incubation period should be known to persons conducting studies like Hahnemann. An infection becomes apparent only after a certain incubation period which is defined as the "time interval between invasion by an infectious agent and appearance of the first sign or symptoms of the disease in question."[248] Infectious agent undergoes multiplication in the host during incubation period. When disease agent becomes insufficient amount, the disease becomes overt. "The factors which determine the incubation period include the generation time of the particular pathogen, infective dose, portal of entry and individual susceptibility.'[249] Incubation period varies for different infectious diseases and this also differs from one patient to another with the same disease.

Incubation period is very short in **cholera**, **bacillary dysentery** and **influenza** *e.g.,* few hours to two to three days. In some diseases it is 10 days to 3 weeks *e.g.,* are **typhoid**, **infection**, **chickenpox**, **measles**, **mumps**. There are also diseases which haveweeks to months or years of incubation period. In these cases, accurate assessment of incubation period is very difficult.

"Non-infectious diseases such as **cancer**, **heart disease** and **mental illness** also have incubation periods which may be months or years."[250]

Now it should be clear in our mind that by only studying symptoms it can never be possible to tell if "one disease cured another similar disease" which is the basic principle of Homeopathy.

32

In Homeopathy "to know effectiveness of a drug, it should not be given to the patients", because in patients symptoms produced by drug and symptoms produced by disease will be mixed and then it will be difficult to separate. To know **therapeutic effectiveness**, drug should be given to healthy persons. In severe acute and chronic diseases which constitute by far the greater portion of all human ailments, crude nature is powerless. In these neither the vital force with its self-aiding faculty nor Allopathy in imitation of it can affect a *lysis.*

ARGUMENT

Natural history of disease should be known to a person who discovers any new treatment. Without knowing the natural course, claim of cure by a drug is useless. The study of the natural course of disease is not a part of any pathy. Normal observation of the natural course of a disease will remain same irrespective of type of pathy. "As wartsoften disappear spontaneously, at any treatment which is in use the time will gain an undeserved reputation as a wart cure."[251]

"Proctitis is an inflammation of rectal mucosa characterized by loss of blood in motions, often the complaint is one of **diarrhoea**, fortunately the condition is self-limiting."[252]

Most viral infections are self-limiting. Typhoid fever is also cured spontaneously when treatment is not given. "The clinical manifestations and duration of illness vary markedly from one patient to another. Mild form of disease characterized primarily by fever may last only for a week or illness may be prolonged lasting upto eight weeks or more if untreated. In a typical patient, not treated with antimicrobials, the illness lasts for about four weeks."[253]

Almost all infectious diseases except few like**rabies** and **HIV**, are spontaneously cured if sufficient immunity is in the body.

"In **diabetic neuropathy**, the most common picture is that of peripheral neuropathy, the symptoms include numbness, **paresthesias**, severe hyperesthesias and pain. The pain which may be deep seated and severe, is often worse at night. Fortunately extreme pain syndromes are usually self-limited.'[254]

Low back pain usually recovers spontaneously. "Low back pain is at epidemic levels. Although its causes are still poorly understood, treatment choices have improved with the body's own healing power often the most reliable remedy. Most back pain patients will substantially and rapidly recover even when their pain is severe. This prognosis holds true regardless of treatment method or even without treatment.'[255]

"In lobar pneumonia in untreated patient resolution occurs on the eighth day. Complete resolution and regeneration take from one to three weeks since there is virtually no tissue destruction in **lobar pneumonia**, the lung parenchyma returns to normal.'[256]

Study of skin diseases play a very important role in the analysis of Homeopathy. According to Homeopathy, suppression of skin diseases by external applications of drugs redirect the diseases internally and creates internal diseases. But, in fact, cure ofskin diseases has no relation with development of internal disease. Many skin diseases are resolved spontaneously which confused Hahnemann who wrongly thought that treatment of skin diseases by external means creates internal pathology. "Various skin diseases tend to recover spontaneously. **Herpes zoster** spontaneously resolves in two to four weeks, chickenpox in two to four weeks; **pityriasis rosacea**, a papulosquamous disease, which recovers in six weeks; **pityriasis** alba—a kind of **eczematous** disorder in which children get **hypopigmented** spots usually disappears after puberty. **Acne vulgaris** usually disappears after the age of 25 years. **Alopecia areata** is the commonest cause of patchy hair loss, is a self-limiting disease. It usually recovers in three to six months. Majority of the cases having **infective dermatoses** also tend to recover even if no treatment is given. Patients having **pyoderma**, **dermatophyte infection** and **candidiasis** tend to improve with the onset of winter without any treatment. **Herpes simplex** usually disappears in one to two weeks but virus may reactivate again in few patients. **Facial warts** may disappear in more than 60 per cent cases without any treatment in three to six months. **Molluscum contagiosum** can disappear in more than 60 per cent cases without treatment in three to six months."[257]

"**Erysipelas**, a specific form of **cellulitis** caused by beta hemolytic streptococci, illustrates the diffusely spreading nature of many streptococci infections.... The lesion is most often self-limited except in the very young or very old."[258]

Carcinomas are malignant tumors and obviously are of clinical importance because of the extensive mortality and morbidity they produce. Most cancers are treated by surgery. Radiotherapy and drug therapy are also part of cancer therapy.

It is the general concept of public that if a person is suffering from cancer he will die or require extensive surgical or non-surgical treatment.

Nobody thinks that cancer may resolve spontaneously but medical reports say that cancer may resolve spontaneously. "Certainly there is an interplay of tumor-host relationship so that all factors combine to determine the ultimate biological behaviour of the neoplasm. Benign tumors not only grow slowly but also at times reach a point where they seem to become dormant or even to regress. This is true *e.g.* with **leiomyomas of the uterus,** which often cease growing after the menopause occasionally even malignant tumors enter a stage of dormancy and in rare but well-documented instances,they may regress spontaneously.'[259]

"In **malignant melanoma** clinically spontaneous regression often heralded by sudden onset of irregular halo around tumour."[260] Tumors are divided into two groups, one is relatively innocuous tumors designated as benign and the other more rapidly growing, dangerous and destructive tumors known as malignant. The synonym ofmalignant tumor is cancer. Benign tumors have no metastases and very little tissue destruction whilc cancer has widespread metastases and much tissue destruction. "**Ganglioneuroma** is a benign tumor of neurological tissue while **neuroblastoma** is a malignant tumor. As a rare but remarkable event

neuroblastoma may undergo a form of self cure by maturing into a **ganglioneuroma**"[261] or may regress spontaneously."[262]

"**Choriocarcinoma** is a highly malignant tumor. In some instances removal of primary tumor has been followed by apparently spontaneous disappearance of metastasis."[263] It is also known to medical science that diseases have a variable natural history. "Most diseases tend to wax and wane in severity, some disappear spontaneously with time, even malignant neoplasm may undergo spontaneous remissions. A good experimental design must take into account the natural history of the disease under study by evaluating a large enough population of subjects over a sufficiently long period of time."[264]

We also know by normal observations that diseases have normal fluctuations. These normal fluctuations and presence of other diseases may influence the result of clinical study. To obtain accurate results "A crossover design which consists of alternating period of administration of test drug, placebo preparation and standard drug control in each subject. These sequences are systemically varied so that different subsets of patients receive each of the possible sequences of treatment."[265]

There is also a psychological effect in patients. Even if an inert material is given to patients, most patients tend to respond in a positive way. It is known as placeboresponse and this may also involve objective biochemical, pathological change and also a change in complaint of patient associated with disease. "The magnitude of the response varies considerably from patient to patient. However, the incidence of the placebo response is fairly constant being observed in 20 to 40 per cent of patients in almost all studies. Placebo toxicity also occurs but usually involves subjective effects in stomach upset, insomnia, sedation."[266] This full method of studying drug clinically is known as double blind placebo controlled crossover design.

"Enormous costs from $100 million to over $500 million (dollar) are involved in the development of a single successful new drug. These costs include the labour invested in searching for useful new molecules. 5000-10000 may be synthesized for each successful new drug introduced and the costs of detailed basic and clinical studies and promotion of the ultimate candidate molecule."[267]

Now we should know how much time will be taken by a drug for its development and what type of studies are required before successful development of a drug or treatment.

Initial safety, biological effects, receptor study, enzyme inhibition and selectivity, drug absorption, metabolism, excretion, therapeutic efficacy, dose range, kinetics and adverse reaction, acute, subacute, chronic studies, effect on reproductive behaviour,carcinogenic potential, **mutagenic** potential are studied and analyzed by clinical **pharmacologist** and physicians.

"Most new drug candidates are identified through chemical modification of known molecule, screening of natural products or previously discovered chemical entities forbiological activity or rational drug design based on an understanding of biological mechanism."[268]

"Average ten years are taken by a drug before marketing'[269] and even after marketing surveillance is continued. If new toxicity appears after marketing drug iswithdrawn from market and the whole exercise of development of drug becomes useless.

Now I am giving only one example of number of patients required for study. "Frequency of myocardial infarction in woman non-smokers 30-39 years of age is about 4 in 100,000. Number of exposed subject required for study is 1800,000.'[270]

Such a vast study, an average 10 years of duration, 500 to 2500 crore rupees are invested in development of a new drug. Conclusively it can be said, "Doctors who think they can assess the value of a treatment by using it on patients in an uncontrolled fashion have the whole history of therapeutics against them."[271]

To know **therapeutic efficacy** of a drug, it should be given to patients and after controlled trials and statistical analysis we can say about effectiveness of a drug or treatment. Drug is given to healthy volunteers to know the pharmacokinetic character and adverse effects of a drug. But in Homeopathy "to know effectiveness of a drug it should not be given to patients because in patients symptoms produced by drug and symptomsproduced by disease will be mixed and then it will be difficult to separate them."[272]

In Homeopathy drug is never studied in patients. Drug is given to healthy persons and symptoms produced by drug are recorded. If the drug produces same symptoms in healthy persons as the disease itself then that drug is considered to be the best treatment for that disease.

Hahnemann was a highly intelligent person but he suffered from lack of accurate information. Capacity to analyse, capacity of invention, creation and research ability indicate intelligence. Knowledge is a collection of information. A highly intelligent person cannot tell the truth if he has wrong information. A highly advanced computer will give wrong conclusion if we feed wrong or incomplete information.

Hahnemann worked during 1810 to 1842. At that time sufficient information regarding health and disease was not available. This is the cause why Hahnemann made wrong conclusions.

Hahnemann said two things very accurately. He should be appreciated for this. First he said that **old Allopathy** is dangerous and detrimental to human body. Hahnemann writes accurately. "Although previously there was never a drop of blood too much in the living human body, yet the old school practitioners consider an imaginary excess of blood as the main material cause of all**haemorrhage** and inflammations which they must remove and drain off by **venesections**, cupping and leeches... . In general inflammatory fevers, in acute pleurisy they even regard the **coagulable** lymph in the blood... . which they endeavor to get rid of if possible by repeated venesections."[273]

"They thus often bleed the patient nearly to death."[274] Second statement which is correctly said by Hahnemann regarding natural recovery of some diseases: "It is only the slighter and acute diseases that tend when the natural period of their course has expired to terminate quietly in resolution, as it is called with or without the employment of not very aggressive allopathic remedies."[275]

Hahnemann agreed that some diseases resolved spontaneously but Hahnemann made the mistake by presuming that severe acute and chronic diseases cannot resolve automatically. As Hahnemann said—

"In severe acute and chronic diseases which constitute by far the greater portion of all human ailments, crude nature and the old school are equally powerless, in these neither the vital force with its self-aiding faculty nor Allopathy in imitation if it, can affect a *lysis*, but at the most a mere temporary truce during which the enemy fortifies himself, in order sooner or later to recommence the attack with still greater violence."[276] It was the biggest mistake made by Hahnemann. Many severe, acute and chronic diseases alsoresolve automatically. This fact was not known to Hahnemann and this is mainly responsible for development of pseudopathy that is Homeopathy.

33

Kent concluded that one chronic disease (**syphilis**) suppressed another chronic disease (**Bright's disease**) and when **syphilis** was cured *Bright's disease* again appeared. Then Kent said—"dissimilar are unable to cure, they can only suppress."

ARGUMENT

Kent's lectures on Homeopathic philosophy have been accepted as authorized documents.

Kent said in his lecture—"A patient is in the earlier stage of **Bright's disease** and the symptoms are clear enough to make a diagnosis. He takes syphilis and at once the kidney disease is held in abeyance, the albumin disappears from the urine and his**waxiness** is lost. But after a year's careful prescribing the syphilitic state disappears and very soon the albumin appears again in the urine, the dropsy returns and he dies of an ordinary attack of **Bright's disease**."[277]

This patient had three stages—

1. Patient suffered with **oedema** and **albuminurea** in first stage which was said to be **Bright's disease**.

2. At the next stage when **syphilis** appeared, **Bright's** disease was cured.
3. In last stage after one year when **syphilis** was resolved, **Bright's disease** again reappeared and patient died. Then Kent said– "dissimilar are unable to cure they can only suppress."[278]

This conclusion that one disease suppresses another dissimilar chronic disease on the basis of above observation was wrong.

What is **Bright's disease**?

"Any one of a group of kidney disease attending with albuminurea and is oedema known as **Bright's** disease."[279] And what are the symptoms of **nephritic syndrome**?

"**Acute nephritic syndrome** consists of the abrupt onset of **hematuria** (reduced G.F.R.) hypertension and edema. Within a week or so of onset most patients with post infectious **acute glomerulonephritis** will begin to experience spontaneous resolution of hypertension and fluid retention."[280]

"In case of **acute post streptococcal glomerulonephritis** all experience a spontaneous resolution of abnormal clinical signs within a week after the onset of illness. Abnormalities in the urinary sediment and protein excretion subside slowly in the ensuing months. In a few cases several years elapse before the urinary sediment becomes consistently normal."[281]

"In many instances **nephritic syndrome** will abate following cure of the infection or withdrawal of the offending medication" [282] and we know that various infections are self-limiting due to body immunity. Today we also know that "**syphilis** itself causes **nephritic syndrome** which is also characterized by albuminuria, hypoalbuminemia and oedema."[283]

And this **nephritic syndrome** is also "included in **Bright's disease**. In secondary **syphilis** renal involvement is associated with proteinuria"[284] "a few patients with **syphilis** develop the **nephritic syndrome**."[285]

Now if we coordinate reference no. 277 to 285 we get the following conclusion:

In reference 277 Kent said that development of syphilis suppresses **Bright's disease** and later on after treatment of syphilis **Bright's disease** reappears and patient dies.

But what was the fact—

The fact was as follows. **Bright's disease** of this patient must have been a part of **secondary syphilis**. First there was an appearance of **Bright's disease** followed by other manifestations of **syphilis**. Some manifestations may dominate in one person while other manifestations may dominate in another person. "The secondary lesions of **syphilis** subside within two to six weeks and the patient enters the latent stage.'[286] After gap of one year there was again appearance of late benign stage of syphilis. In this stage **gumma** is produced which may be multiple or diffuse. By **gumma** "any organ may be involved and about one-fourth die as a result of tertiary syphilis"[287] or in Kent's observation in reference no. 277 the earlier part of disease must have been a type of **Bright's disease** which was cured spontaneously as mentioned in reference nos. 280 and 281. And the second and third part of disease was definitely secondary and tertiary stage of syphilis. Patient died due to kidney lesions of tertiary syphilis. Now we can say that by only studying symptoms and without studying other aspects of disease and without proper diagnosis and evaluation nothing can be said. If somebody says empirically then it will be definitely incorrect as Kent and Hahnemann said.

34

Homeopathy **condemns** the principle of the **removal** of **external manifestations** of disease by external means whatsoever.

ARGUMENT

"Homeopathy condemns the principle of the removal of external manifestations of disease by external means whatsoever."[288] For the support of this statement Kent gives the example of **fistula in ano**. Kent writes—"the closure of that fistulous opening of the anus will throw him into a flame of excitement and will cause his death in a year or two. The fistulous opening came there because it was useful. When the patient is cured the fistulous opening ceases to be of use, the necessity for it to remain open has ceased and it heals up of itself."[289]

Generalization should not have been made by Kent and Hahnemann from single or a few observations. External outlet is a must where pus is collected. Pus should be removed. If pus is not removed then it is very difficult to get cured.

In **fistula in ano** "The **fistula** continues to discharge and because of constant reinfection from the canal or rectum, seldom if ever close permanently without surgical aid."[290]

Kent also writes—"If a patient is threatened with **phthisis** or is a weakly patient, closure of fistulous opening of the anus will cause his death."[291]

Today we know "about two to three per cent of **fistula in ano** patient are **tuberculous.** The **fistula** will usually respond to antitubercular drug."[292] **Fistula in ano** has varied **aetiology** like **tuberculosis, ulcerative proctocolitis, Crohn's disease, bilharziasis, lymphogranuloma inguinale,** etc. This varied **aetiology** and continuous contamination and accumulation of pus requires evacuation of pus and treatment of specific cause.

But generalization should not be made that external symptoms should not be managed.

Homeopathy does not accept the concept of externally localized independent disease. According to this pathy all localized external lesions are actually parts of internal disease. This pathy also opposes treatment of external lesions by external means. When localized lesion is a part of generalized internal disease then in such case external localized treatment may not be effective. Internal disease has to be treated *e.g.* **syphilis, gonorrhoea**. But when external lesions are not parts of generalized disease then external management has to be used. Today we know various diseases which are externally localized lesions and these are not parts of internal generalized diseases.

These are treated effectively by external means. Following are examples: "Cyst, sinuses, sebaceous cyst, **papilloma** of skin, **molluscum fibrosum, molluscum sebaceum,** basal cell carcinoma of the skin, **squamous** cell carcinoma of skin, **chalazion**, cataract, conjunctivitis, cleft lip, cleft palate, **neoplasms** of the lip, boils, carbuncle, **hyperplastic** ingivitis, neoplasm of the breast, etc., are the pathological lesions which can be managed only by external localized means. These lesions are independent and localized."[293]

In above examples **external manifestations** are removed by **external therapeutic methods** which indicates Homeopathic concept of opposition of external treatment is wrong.

35

No organ can make the body **sick**. Man is **prior** to his **organs**. Parts of the body can be removed and yet man will **exist**.

ARGUMENT

Kent writes—

"Hahnemann, it seems would say that it is great folly for a man to look into the organs themselves for the purpose of establishing a theory to find out whether the stomach makes the man sick or whether the stomach makes the liver sick and such like."[294]

Kent also writes—

"No organ can make the body **sick**, man is **prior** to his **organs**, parts of the body can be removed and yet man will **exist**. There is no such thing as one organ making another sick."[295]

Kent says no organ can make the body sick but what is reality?

"**Delirium** is characterized by clouding of consciousness perceptual disturbances, incoherent speech, altered psychomotor activity disorientation and memory impairment."[296] This means a person suffering from **delirium** indicates sickness. And **delirium** is produced by pathology of specific organ. "Pathology in brain, pituitary, pancreas, adrenal gland, parathyroid and thyroid glands liver, kidney, lung, heart can produce **delirium**. Any one of the above organs can develop **delirium** when pathology occurs in that part."[297]

Body can become sick when lung or liver or heart or kidney or any other organ of the body is damaged. Liver disorder creates **hepatic coma**. **Kidney failure** is responsible for death. **Heart failure** also damages the whole body. **Heart attack** is the main cause of death. When pathology or disease in one organ can cause death then how can Kent say that damage or disease of one organ cannot make the body sick. Now we can say that this statement of Kent is also wrong.

Kent further says that parts of body can be removed and yet man will exist. How a man can survive when his liver or heart or both lungs or both kidneys or brain are removed. A man can never survive when his vital organs are removed. Only a brainless person can say that a man can survive without a brain. Kent also said—"One organ cannot make another organ sick."

But the whole medical knowledge says that one damaged organ always damages the other organ. I am giving few examples—

1. **Chronic obstructive lung disease** is a disease of lung. After sometime this disease damages the heart which is known as **cor pulmonale**.
2. **Cancer** of one organ affects various organs of body by **matastasis.** For example, "Carcinoma in kidney affects adrenal gland, bone, brain, heart, lung, liver, lymph node, ovary, pancreas, skin, spleen thyroid gland and muscles."[298] Similarly cancer of many organs can affect other organs of body.
3. Disease of pancreas gives rise to **diabetes mellitus**. **Diabetes** of prolonged duration damages kidney, eye and nervous system.
4. Damage in the brain also causes damage to other organs of body. Brain controls all the functions of body. Damage in brain leads to **hemiplegia**, **paraplegia**, vision loss, speech loss, etc. **Hemiplegia** means paralysis of half of body and **paraplegia** means paralysis of both the lower limbs.

Conclusively, Kent was again wrong in his observations.

36

How did Hahnemann reach the conclusion that it is not the external cause that a man becomes sick, neither bacteria, nor environment but the causes are in himself. He said **intravenous administration** of fluid is **dangerous** to body and bacteria have not been sent on earth to destroy man. Bacteria are perfectly **harmless** in every respect.

ARGUMENT

Kent and Hahnemann say again and again "It is not from external things that man becomes sick, not from bacteria nor environment but from causes in himself."[299]

Hahnemann derived this conclusion on the basis of some results mentioned by some contemporary experts:

(1) "A girl in Glasgow eight years of age having been bit by a mad dog, the surgeon immediately cut the piece clean out and yet 36 days afterwards she was seized with **hydrophobia** which killed her in two days."[300]

(2) "Life was endangered by injecting a little pure water into a vein."
(3) "Even the mildest fluids introduced into the vein endangered life."[301]

In example one Hahnemann observed that after dog bite, although part was cleaned and removed from the body the patient suffered from **hydrophobia** and died. That's why he concluded that external micro-organism was not responsible for **hydrophobia** and death. Then he presumed that cause of **hydrophobia** was within the person and not related with dog bite. Truth was missed by Hahnemann. Reality was as follows: "**Rabies** also known as **hydrophobia**, is an acute and highly fatal viral disease of the central nervous system. It is transmitted to man usually by bites or licks of rabid animals. **Rabies** virus spreads from the site of infection centripetally via the peripheral nerves towards thecentral nervous system, most likely it ascends passively through the nerve associated tissue space. Bite wounds should not be immediately sutured to prevent additional trauma which may help spread the virus into the deeper tissues."[302]

In this example dissection at the site of dog bite exposed nerve endings which facilitated virus transmission to the central nervous system. "Once the virus reaches the central nervous system, it replicates almost exclusively within the grey matter and then passes centrifugally along autonomic nerves to reach other tissue'[303] and causes death. In example two, Hahnemann studied observations of other physician and found that intravenous administration of fluid is dangerous to body. But this observation was absolutely wrong. Today drugs and fluid are routinely administered intravenously and lives of crores of patients are saved. **Cefotaxim**, **ampicillin**, **gentamycin**, **ciprofloxacin**, **metronidazole**, **aminophyllin**, **corticosteroids**, **morphine derivatives**, **electrolytes**, water and saline are also administered intravenously and patients get benefitted. Intravenous administration of substance is not dangerous to life.

Regarding air administration Hahnemann's opinion was correct. Air administration in circulation is dangerous to life and may cause death.

All substances cannot be administered intravenously, it is correct. Intravenous route increased risk of adverse effects. It is not suitable for oily solutions. Drug should be in aqueous solution to administer by intravenous route. Insoluble substances, if administered by intravenous route, damage the body and may cause death.

In the above examples Hahnemann wanted to say, "The causes of our maladies cannot be material since the least foreign material substance, however mild it may appear to us, if introduced into our blood vessels is

promptly ejected by vital force, as though it were a poison or when this does not happen death ensues."[304] But conclusion of Hahnemann was wrong and observations of respective physicians were also wrong who said intravenous fluid administration caused death.

Kent also writes—

"The bacteria are results of disease. **Microscopical** little fellows are not the disease cause but they come after that. They are scavengers accompanying the disease and that they are perfectly harmless in every respect. They are the outcome of the disease, are present wherever the disease is and by the microscope it has been discovered that every pathological result has its corresponding bacteria."[305]

Kent also writes—

"Bacteria have a use for there is nothing in the whole world that does not have a use and there is nothing sent on earth to destroy man. The bacteria theory would make it appear that the all wise creator has sent these micro-organisms here to make man sick. Hahnemann did not adopt any such theory as bacteriology."[306]

Kent also writes—

"Cause of **phthisis** not in the bacteria but in the virus which the bacteria are sent to destroy. Man lives longer with the bacteria than he would without them."[307] Today it has been proved that bacteria are the causes of so many diseases like **tuberculosis**, **leprosy**, **typhoid**, **dysentery**, **meningitis**, **gonorrhoea**, respiratory tract infection, etc. If somebody still accepts the view that bacteria are not responsible for any disease, then we can say that he does not know anything regarding medical science. Same statement is true for those who believe in Homeopathy.

In support of the view that bacteria are not responsible for any disease, Kent writes—

"A dissecting wound is very serious if the body dissected is recently dead and this we would suppose to be due to some bacteria of wonderful power capable of establishing such dreadful **erysipelatous** poisoning that would go into man's blood and strike him down with a sort of **septicaemia**. In truth, soon after death we have a **ptomaine** poison, the dead body poison, which is alkaloid in character but we do not yet discover the presence of bacteria. The poison is there and if a man pricks himself while dissecting that body and does not take care of the wound he may have a serious illness and die. But ifafter the cadaver has remained sometime and become infected with bacteria, the dissector pricks himself and the wound is not dangerous."[308]

Kent did not agree that **erysipelas** infection was due to bacteria. The Kent was of the opinion that after death there is production of **ptomaine** poison in dead body which is fatal to living being and bacteria are not related with production of this **ptomaine poison**. Kent also said that after death, body was infected with bacteria but these bacteria were not harmful to body because bacteria from cadaver did not make the wound dangerous.

All these conclusions of Kent were wrong. It has been proved today that "**Erysipelas** is an acute infection of the skin and subcutaneous tissue caused by group A streptococci, other streptococci and even staphylococci and pneumococci."[309] All these organisms are bacteria and responsible for **erysipelas diseases**. Kent did not know regarding **ptomaine** poison how it is produced and in what amount it is dangerous. Today we know "**Ptomains** are **alkaloidal** bodies produced by the action of saprophytic micro-organisms upon nitrogenous materials, probably during the process of decomposition. They are called **cadaveric** alkaloids as they are generated in the dead tissue while alkaloids secreted by the living cells during the metabolic processes are called **leucomaines**. Most of the **ptomains** that have been discovered are non-poisonous except **neurine** and **mydaleine**, which are actively poisonous and produce symptoms resembling those produced by **atropine**, **muscarine, aconite**. It is said that **neurine** is not generated till the fifth or sixth day has elapsed since death and **mydaleine** not until the seventh day and that too in traces only."[310]

Usually **ptomains** are of two types only—non-poisonous and poisonous. The poisonous **ptomains** are produced in very small amounts and by dissecting instrument the amount which is transferred from dead body to living tissue is very very less and less likely to produce toxic **symptomatology** in healthy persons. **Ptomains** are produced by bacteria. Again Kent was wrong about statement which he gave for **ptomains**.

Kent also writes that bacteria present in cadaver are not harmful and because they do not make wound dangerous that's why Kent makes conclusion that bacteria cannot produce any disease or do any harm to human being. But Kent was always wrong. He could not understand the facts due to lack of available knowledge. Why bacteria from cadaver cannot produce disease in healthy human being? The answer is as follows:

"Clostridium welchi, Clostridium oedematiens and Clostridium septicum are three most important anaerobic sporulatingbacteria. Being anaerobic and saprophytic, they cannot multiply in living, oxygenated tissue but they flourish in dead tissue. The dead tissues are commonly invaded by a mixture of other organisms which may play a major role in putrefaction."[311]

The bacteria which usually grows in dead tissue are anaerobic which cannot grow and multiply in living tissue because of oxygen.

Oxygen interferes growth and multiplicationof these anaerobic bacteria. That's why bacteria growing in dead tissue are not harmful to living tissue. "It has been learned that the intense oxidizing properties of high pressure oxygen (**hyperbaric** oxygen) can have valuable therapeutic effects in several important clinical conditions, probably the most successful use of **hyperbaric** oxygen has been in the treatment of gas gangrene. The bacteria that cause this condition **clostridial** organisms, grow best under anaerobic conditions and stop growing at oxygen pressure greater than about 70 m.m. Hg. Therefore, **hyperbaric** oxygenation of the tissues can frequently stop the infectious process entirely and this converts a condition that formerly was almost 100 per cent fatal into one that is cured in most instance."[312]

Whenever tissue oxygenation is less or blocked by some interference in blood supply these saprophytic micro-organisms grow in the body and produce disease.

"The most important prerequisite for the conversion of**clostridial** contamination of a wound to a progressive infection is an environment with low oxidation reduction potential, which permits spore germination and anaerobic growth. Local oxidation reduction potential can be reduced by failure of the blood supply to a contaminated areaor by multiplication of other bacteria in the wound. Once multiplication and toxinproduction are established rapid invasion and destruction of healthy tissue follows."[313]

Now it is clear why bacteria from dead body cannot produce disease in healthy tissue but when tissue oxygenation is reduced, these saprophytic micro-organisms become dangerous to body. Now again we can write that concept of Kent is wrong regarding bacteria and disease.

There is no necessity of giving explanation of all examples which had been used by Hahnemann. Explanation of few examples is sufficient.

Hahnemann and Kent could not understand the reality and framed false Homeopathic rules. I am giving one more example, Hahnemann saw "The slightest breath of air emitting from the body of a person affected with smallpox will suffice to produce this horrible disease in healthy child"[314] then Hahnemann said, "who can prove that some material portion of this substance has penetrated into our fluids or been absorbed."[315]

In this example Hahnemann did not know that smallpox is due to virus and which can spread by air inhalation. "Direct transmission for short distance occurs through projection of droplets or droplet nuclei from the upper respiratory tract of an infected host."[316]

Hahnemann did not know that virus can transmit via respiratory route that's why he was not able to understand how disease material can penetrate into body and cause diseases. So he never accepted external material as a disease agent.

Micro-organisms are not the only aetiology for diseases. There are various diseases in which micro-organisms are never responsible. Genetics and internal factors are also responsible for many diseases. **Hypertension**, **cardiac problems**, **carcinomas**, **diabetes**, **endocrinological abnormalities**, **gastric ulcers**, **arthritis**, **immunological diseases**, **schizophrenia, mania** are various examples where external material substance is not entered into the body.

37

Hahnemann **criticized** derivation, imitation and counter-imitation by saying "it is unhelpful, injurious and indirect mode of treatment." He also **opposed** large doses which were being used by old Allopaths.

ARGUMENT

It has been observed that "The degenerated substances and impurities that appear in diseases are undeniably nothing more than the products of disease, if the abnormally deranged organism which are expelled by the latter often violently enough... .Nature assists the diseased organism, resolves fever by perspiration, other diseases by vomiting, **diarrhoea** and bleeding from the anus, **articular** pains by suppurating ulcers of legs."[317]

By observing nature, "old school of medicine thought the best thing to do was to imitate nature, by means of stronger heterogeneous irritants applied to organs remote from the seat of disease and totally dissimilar to the affected tissues, they produce evacuations and generally kept them up in order to draw as it were the disease thither. In this imitation they endeavoured to excite by force new symptoms in the tissues that are least diseased."[318] "To assist this derivative method, old school of medicine employed the allied treatment by counter irritants, woollen garments to the bare skin, foot baths, nauseant, substances to cause pain, inflammation and suppuration in near or distant parts as the application of horseradish, *mustard plasters*, canthrides, **btisters, mezereum setons**, issues, *tartar emetic*, ointments, moxa actual cautery, acupuncture, etc. by exciting pain in distant parts of body or by metastases and abscess by eruptions and suppurating ulcers."[319]

Hahnemann rightly criticized this mode of treatment. I have said many times that Hahnemann opposed the old school of medicine, not present advanced medical science. Hahnemann opposed derivation, imitation and counter-irritation by saying that "It is unhelpful and injurious indirect mode of treatment. The derivatives as well as the counter-irritant thatled them to this inefficacious debilitating and hurtful practice of apparently ameliorating disease for a short time or removing them in such a manner that another and a worse disease was roused up to occupy the place of the first. Such a destructive plan cannot certainly be termed curing."[320]

Hahnemann opposed old school of medicine due to some other reasons also. Old Allopaths had been using drugs in very large doses.

"*Cinchona bark* was being used for all epidemic intermittent *fevers* with enormous doses of *cinchona* and its costly alkaloid quinine. He deluded patient become worse then he was during the fever itself."[321]

Similarly due to large dose of "*Digitalis* **purpurea**... . sleep, appetite and strength of patient are lost, death is imminent, not one of the patients so treated escapes alive, unless to be a prey to incurable insanity."[322]

Hahnemann criticized the old school of medicine rightly by saying: "Mixture in a prescription of various medicinal substances whose real action was almost without an exception, unknown.... The result naturally belies every expectation that had been formed. They certainly ensue changes and results but none of an appropriate character, non-beneficial, all injurious destructive old school knows not what else to do with patients suffering from chronic diseases than to attack the sufferers with drugs that do nothing but torture them, waste their strength and fluids and shorten their lives."[323]

Conclusively, it can be said that Hahnemann's criticism of old school of medicine or old Allopathy was correct. The concept and methodology of old school of medicine can never be correlated with modern advanced medical science. Old school of medicine was not accurate. Today we are able to say with certainty that Homeopathy is also wrong.

38

It is only the slighter and acute disease that tend to terminate quietly in resolution or in death. All chronic diseases of mankind cannot be cured spontaneously. These evermore increase with the years. They never pass away on their own but keep increasing and are aggravated even till death. There are three chronic diseases (1) **Syphilis**, (2) **Sycosis**, and (3) **Psora**.

ARGUMENT

Now it is being analyzed here how Hahnemann, Kent and their followers made mistakes. The most important part of discovery of therapeutics is knowledge of normal course and normal process of disease when external therapeutic measures are not provided. Without knowing the normal course of disease, it is totally useless to claim successful treatment of disease.

All diseases are not always fatal. Today **AIDS** is a fatal disease. Once a person is infected with **AIDS** virus, he will definitely die. Nothing can save him.

Many diseases have spontaneous cure. Tropical diseases are usually resolved spontaneously. Tropical diseases mean diseases originated due to external infective agents and transmitted usually by dirty water, dirty food and unhygienic surroundings.

By treatment, course of disease is shortened, intensity of symptomatology is reduced, morbidity and mortality are also lessened.

But to know such importance of treatment comparative study with control is a must. Without doing comparative and therapeutic trials, we cannot establish utility of a treatment. If a disease is going to be resolved spontaneously and somebody says, "This cure is due to my treatment" then it is a foolish comment. Same mistakes were made by Hahnemann and Kent and by their followers. They did not study normal course of the diseases and blindly claimed that they were able to cure many chronic diseases by their Homeopathic remedies.

Hahnemann divided diseases into two groups. "The diseases to which man is liable are either rapid morbid processes of the abnormally deranged vital force, which have a tendency to finish their course more or less quickly, but always in a moderate time these are termed acute diseases."[324]

Hahnemann further writes—

"It is only the slighter and acute diseases that tend when the natural period of their course has expired, to terminate quietly in resolution as it is called with or without the employment of not very aggressive allopathic remedies, vital force having regained its power, then gradually substitutes the normal condition for the derangement of the health that has now ceased to exist."[325]

Hahnemann also writes—

"Allied to these (acute disease) are those diseases in which many persons are attacked with very similar sufferings from the same cause (epidemically); these diseasesgenerally become infectious (contagious) when they prevail among thickly congregated masses of human beings. Thence arise fevers in each instance of a peculiar nature and because the cases of disease have an identical origin, they set up in all those they affect an identical morbid process which when left to itself terminates in a moderate period time in death or recover."[326]

Now it is clear by the above writing that Hahnemann was of opinion that some acute diseases are resolved spontaneously without any external treatment.

Hahnemann raised question against the old school of medicine rightly—

"It remains a very doubtful question whether the natural process of recovery in acute diseases is really at all shortened or facilitated by this interference of the old school, as the latter cannot act otherwise than the vital force, namely indirectly, but its derivative and counter irritant treatment is much more injurious and much more debilitating."[327]

The objection of Hahnemann was right against old school of medicine because no controlled study was done and normal course of the disease was also not known to old school of medicine. Same questions can also be raised against Homeopathy when treatment of chronic diseases are concerned. Hahnemann knew this fact that some acute diseases are resolved spontaneously without any treatment. For this Hahnemann should be appreciated. When question of chronic diseases arises, Hahnemann was also wrong.

Hahnemann writes regarding chronic diseases—

"They are diseases of such a character that with small often imperceptible beginnings, dynamically derange the living organism, each in its peculiar manner, and cause it gradually to deviate from the healthy condition in such a way that the automatic life energy called vital force, whose office is to preserve the health only opposes them at the commencement and during their process imperfect unsuitable, useless resistance but is unable of itself to extinguish them but helplessly suffer itself to be ever more and more abnormally deranged until at length the organism is destroyed, these are termed chronic diseases."[328]

Hahnemann also writes—

"All chronic diseases of mankind even those left to themselves.... They evermore increase with the years and during the whole of man's lifetime and they cannot be diminished by the strength belonging even to the most robust constitution.... They never pass away of themselves but increase and are aggravated even till death. The chronic diseases... first **syphilis** which I have also called the general chancre disease, then **sycosis** or **figwart disease** and finally the chronic disease which lies at the foundation of the eruption of itch **psora... psora** is the oldest miasmatic chronic disease known to us. Just as tedious as **syphilis** and **sycosis** and therefore not to be extinguished before the last breath of the longest human life, unless it is thoroughly cured, since not even the most robust constitution is able to destroy and extinguish it by its own proper strength."[329]

It was also said by Hahnemann, "In severe acute and chronic diseases which constitute by far the greatest portion of all human ailments crude nature and the old school are equally powerless."[330]

In these paragraphs, Hahnemann wanted to say that chronic diseases are not able to resolve spontaneously. For the treatment of chronic diseases drugs have to be given. Hahnemann treated chronic diseases by drugs and he got the results. He thought that he was curing the disease by drugs. But, in fact, the chronic diseases, treated by Hahnemann were resolved spontaneously. He did not know this fact. He thought erroneously that his drugs were effective in treating chronic diseases and he wrongly formulated law of Homeopathy. Hahnemann had a misconception that— "True natural chronic diseases are those that arise from a chronic miasm... always go on increasing and growing worse, notwithstanding the best mental and corporeal regimen and torment the patient to the end of his life with ever aggravated suffering. These, excepting those produced by medical malpractice are the most numerous and greatest scourges of the human race; for the most robust constitution, the best regulated mode of living and the most vigorous energy of the vital force are insufficient for their eradication."[331]

39

Syphilis alone has been to some extent known as such a chronic miasmatic disease which when uncured ceases only with the termination of life.

ARGUMENT

Hahnemann mentioned causes of diseases. They are only three according to him **psora, syphilis** and **sycosis**. Cause of acute diseases are "transient explosion of latent **psora** which spontaneously returns to its dormant state if the acute diseases were not of too violent a character and were soon quelled."[332] Causes of chronic disease according to Homeopaths are **psora**, **syphilis** and **sycosis**. **Syphilis** mainly confused Hahnemann, Kent and their followers. **Syphilis** is one of the main diseases which is responsible for development of Homeopathy.

Hahnemann writes—

"Syphilis alone has been to some extent known as such a chronic miasmatic disease, which when uncured ceases only with the termination of life."[333]

Hahnemann did not know actual aetiology, pathogenesis and prognosis of **syphilis** and other sexually transmitted diseases. There are five main sexually transmitted diseases. These are **gonorrhoea**, **syphilis**, **chancroid**, **lymphogranuloma venereum** and **granuloma inguinal**. There are also other diseases having bacterialviral, protozoal, fungal aetiology which might be considered sexually transmitted diseases, with twenty three sexually transmitting pathogens. For diagnosis and detection of specific aetiological agents by microscope and serological testing are very much important otherwise diagnosis is very difficult. Hahnemann did not accept external micro-organism as aetiology that's why at the time of Hahnemann it was not possible to diagnose specific sexually transmitted disease. As mentioned in history of medicine"The erroneous concept that **gonorrhoea**, **chancroid** and **syphilis** were the same disease was strengthened by John Hunter, who developed **syphilis** following self inoculation with **gonorrhoea** pus in 1767. These three diseases were finally distinguished in the mid-1800s, although their aetiologies were not established until the turn of this century. Gummas were not recognized as being **syphilitic** in origin until this century. The discovery of Treponema pallidum in serum from secondary lesion was made by Schaudinn in 1905 and was confirmed by Landsteiner in 1906. Wasserman introduced the complete fixation test for the diagnosis of **syphilis** in the same year."[334]

And this information should be kept in mind by readers that Hahnemann did his work during 1800 to 1850.

Now we are concentrating ourselves in the comparative analytical study of **syphilis**. We will compare the information regarding **syphilis** which were present at the time of Hahnemann and what we have today.

I have written previously that—

Hahnemann presumed **syphilis** cannot be resolved spontaneously. Homeopathic drugs have to be given for the treatment of **syphilis**.

But today by normal observations of **syphilitic** patients without giving any treatment we have found that many patients were cured spontaneously. Little knowledge of **syphilis** is necessary to understand the facts of Homeopathy. "**Syphilis**"[335] is a chronic infection due to **Trepanoma pallidum.** It is systemic from the beginning, runs a chronic course characterized by florid features at sometimes but by long periods of latency at other times. It may be latent throughout and its course is variable. After an incubation period of 9 to 90 days ***the primary lesion*** or **chancre** develops at the site of infection usually on the genitalia. A small pink macule appears which becomes, papular and ulcerate. The primary **chancre** heals and six to eight weeks later malaise, headache and fever appear. Four signs appear—a rash, **lymphadenopathy, condylomata** and mucous patches—though any ofthem may be absent. **Condylomata** are large flat papules which develop around the anus, rarely eye, joints, bone or abdominal viscera, nervous system may be affected. After several months the ***secondary changes*** gradually disappear to be followed by a latent period.

Latency may persist for many years. ***Tertiary stage*** takes 10 or more years to develop and affects skin, mucous membrane, subcutaneous tissue, submucosa, long bone mainly. The characteristic finding is called gumma. Lesions run a long benign course. In the ***quaternary stage*** there are two main conditions—one is **cardiovascular syphilis** and second is **neurosyphilis**.

These usually take longer to develop morbidity and may lead to the patients death. These stages develop after 15 to 20 years of primary infection.

Now we should know normal prognosis of **syphilitic** patients when treatment is not being given. Medical observations say—

"Following the secondary stage untreated adults fall into four groups (a) One-third remain symptomless throughout life with a persistent positive W.R. (Wassermann reaction—an antigen antibody reaction), (b) One-third are likewise symptomless, with a W.R. which ultimately becomes negative, (c) One-sixth develop early tertiary symptoms which abort spontaneously, (d) One-sixth develop and suffer from disease affecting many different systems of the body. The first two groups are termed as **latent syphilis**. It is not possible to know beforehand whether the disease will remain latent or whether it will cause future complications in some vital part."[336]

In another study it has been found—

"The primary lesion appears at the site of inoculation persists for 2 to 6 weeks and then heals spontaneously. Some patients enter the latent stage without ever developing secondary lesions. The secondary lesions subside within 2 to 6 weeks and the patient enters the latent stage, which is detectable only by serological testing. About one-third of patients with untreated **latent syphilis** develop clinically apparent tertiary disease."[337]

"Oslo study and Tuskegee study show that about one-third of patients with untreated **syphilis** develop clinical or pathological evidence of **tertiary syphilis,** about one-fourth die as a direct result of tertiary **syphilis**."[338]

By analysing results of normal prognosis of **syphilitic** patients, it can be concluded that 60 to 70 per cent of **syphilitic** patients are cured spontaneously without giving any treatment. The another important aspect of **syphilis is**—"The average interval from infection to onset of symptoms is 5 to 10 years for **meningovascular syphilis**, 20 years for general **paresis** and 25 to 30 years for **tabes dorsalis**."

Twenty to thirty per cent of **syphilitic** patients develop neurological or cardiovascular complications. But development of these complications take long time of 5 to 30 years.Observation of patients up to 30 years would not have been possible at the time of Hahnemann and Kent.

Sixty to seventy percent of **syphilitic** patients are cured spontaneously and remaining patients take very long time to develop complications. After short time observations it can beconcluded wrongly that all **syphilitic** patients have been cured by any treatment which has been given to such patients. These mistakes definitely have been made by Hahnemann and Kent. They provided useless Homeopathic treatment to **syphilitic** patients and concluded wrongly that they had cured **syphilis**. This conclusion, we canverify by further analysis as follows—

Hahnemann writes, "The **chancre** appears after an impure coition usually between the seventh and fourteenth days first as a little pustule which changes into an impure ulcer with raised borders and stinging pains which if not cured remains standing in the same place during a man's lifetime, only increasing with years while the secondary symptoms of the venereal disease, **syphilis** cannot break out as long as it exists."[340]

Hahnemann agreed with this statement that **syphilis** always follows the destruction of the chancre by local application. Hahnemann also writes, "I have never in my practice of more than fifty years seen any trace of venereal disease break out, so long as the chancre remained untouched in its place even if this were a space of several years for it never passes away of itself and even it had largely increased itsplace."[341]

Today we know regarding **syphilis** that **primary chancre** heals spontaneously and six to eight weeks later secondary symptoms appear irrespective of external manipulation of **chancre**. Systemic manifestation of **syphilis** is not related with destruction or some sort of external treatment of **chancre**. If **chancre** remains for a prolonged time then definitely it is not **syphilis**, it is something else. In to my opinion, Hahnemann was not able to differentiate between **chancre** and **chancroid.** He wrongly labelled **chancroid** and told them chancre. Actually they were **chancroid** not chancre.

"**Chancroid** or soft **chancre** is sexually transmitted infection characterized by painful genital ulceration. **Haemophilus ducreyi** is the cause which is a bacterium. Theincidence of **chancroid** is unknown owing to inaccurate clinical diagnosis and incomplete reporting. Prostitution plays a major role in transmission and among merchants, seaman and military troops whose sexual contacts are prostitutes, **chancroid** is more common than **syphilis**. In contrast to **syphilis** the **chancroidal** ulcer in males is painful and not indurated. Acute, painful tender inflammatory inguinal **adenopathy** occurs in almost 50 per cent of patients and frequently unilateral. The involved nodes become matted forming a unilocular suppurative bubo. The overlying skin becomes erythematous and tense and finally rupture forming a deep single ulcer. **Chancroid** rarely causes systemic symptoms. The **chancre** of primary **syphilis** is indurated and the associated adenopathy is bilateral, non-tender and non-suppurative. Untreated **chancroidal** ulcers persist for long period of time and often progress. Small lesions may heal within two to four weeks."[342]

Hahnemann described **syphilitic chancre** that "it has been substituted by a far more painful substitute the bubo which hastens onward to suppuration."[343]

This indicates clearly that Hahnemann confused **syphilitic chancre** with **chancroid.** He was not able to differentiate between these two and **chancroid** is also a self-limiting disease as mentioned in medical science today.

"**Chancroid** (**Soft chancre**) is an acute: specific, localized self-limiting autoinoculable infectious disease almost always acquired through sexual contact. During medieval times **chancroid** was not distinguished from the initial lesion of **syphilis**. **Gonorrhoea** and **syphilis** were differentiated about 1831, but it was not until 1850 that soft **chancre** was distinguished from the initial lesion of **syphilis** and later designated **chancroid** (**chancre like**). The ulcers of **chancroid** are painful containing pus and may rupture spontaneously. Most commonly the disease is self limiting but in some cases with relatively prolong disability and tissue destruction may ensue."

40

Hahnemann writes regarding treatment of **syphilis** that it needs only one little dose of the best mercurial remedy in order to cure thoroughly and forever the whole ***syphilis*** with its *chancre* within fourteen days. He also used arsenic in the treatment of ***syphilis*** in single dose.

ARGUMENT

"In the past, *potassium iodide*, *mercury*, *bismuth* and *organic arsenical* compounds were used in **syphilis**. Mercury was originally used for **syphilis** but was superseded by *bismuth* and *arsphenamines*."[345] These metallic compounds are highly toxic to body that's why they are not used nowadays. They have been replaced by antibiotics today.

When *mercury* was being used in the treatment of **syphilis** by oral route, "the medication had been administered several times a day for a long period of time. The *protoiodide of mercury* in dose of 1/5 to 1/2 grain was probably the most commonly administered salt. It is powerful containing 61 per cent of the metal but it is very liable to causeintestinal irritation and **diarrhoea**. *Mercury* with chalk in dose of 1 to 3 grains or the **tannate** of mercury in 1/2 to 1 grain dose were appropriate forms of medication. Injection of soluble mercurial salts were also used for a long period of time."[346]

Regarding injectable *mercurial compounds* in treatment of **syphilis** it has been mentioned in medical literature, "In the first case a soluble *mercurial salt* is thrown almost directly into the blood giving an immediate most vigorous therapeutic effect but one, which if that action is to be sustained, it requires repetition of medication everyday. Objective symptoms as skin eruption and ulcerative lesion begin to improve in a day or two. It is the subjective symptoms however that show the therapeutic effect of injections most brilliantly. Improvement in general feeling begins in a few hours. Symptomsdisappear and lesions heal with rapidity. The usually single parental dose of *mercury* compound was 0.065 gram."[347]

Mercury should be administered in compound form. Doses which were used by Hahnemann are as follows—

"Hahnemann writes, in **syphilis**, it needs only one little dose of the best mercurial remedy in order to cure thoroughly and forever the whole **syphilis** with its chancre within fourteen days. He formerly used the billionth dynamization (ii) of this preparation, although the preparation of the higher potency (iv, vi, viii) and finally the **decillionth** potency show some advantages in their quick penetrating and yet mild action for this purpose, but in cases where a second or third dose (however seldom needed) should be found necessary a lower potency then be taken."[348]

Hahnemann himself writes regarding potency of drug—"The material part of the medicine is lessened with each degree of **dynamization** 50000 times.... The 30th thus progressively prepared would give a fraction almost impossible to be expressed in numbers."[349]

"The degree of dynamization are frequently so expressed that only the exponent showing how often 100 has been multiplied into itself is expressed."[350]

Above description shows that one decillion dilution means 10^{60} dilution, which is equal to thirtieth potency. One gram drug is dissolved into 10^{60} ml. of water or alcohol then it will be equal to 30th potency we can say that such dilution will not contain any drug molecule. How drug of this dilution with one dose only can cure a disease? On other hand mercury compounds in doses of 0.065 gms, many times a day for prolonged period was being given for treatment of **syphilis**. We can say, Homeopathic drug means no drug. It is just placebo.

The positive results claimed by Homeopathic drugs are actually result of the spontaneous cure.

Hahnemann committed one more mistake. When external **chancre** remained localized and resolved spontaneously or remained localized without systemic manifestations, Hahnemann said it was **syphilis** which had been cured by antisyphilitic drug.

Here Hahnemann was wrong. It was actually **chancroid** which usually never gives systemic manifestations, remains localized or cure spontaneously.

If systemic manifestations of **syphilis** were present, Hahnemann thought, "He can cure these patients by antipsoric drug in addition to antisyphilitic drug." In the view of Hahnemann, systemic manifestations of **syphilis** was due to **psora**. Here again he was wrong. Actually systemic manifestations of secondary stage of **syphilis** heal spontaneously. This healing was not due to antipsoric drug advised by Hahnemann, but he thought wrongly. He writes—

"**Psora** which had as yet been latent within him has been brought to its development and has broken out into chronic ailments and these irrepressibly combine with the **internal syphilis**."[351]

Regarding false belief of curing **syphilis** Master and Johnson write clearly—

"The **chancre** generally appears two to four weeks after infection, **chancre** is painless in 75 per cent of cases. The **chancre** usually heals within four to six weeks, leading to the erroneous belief that the problem went away. **Secondary syphilis** begins anywhere from one week to six months after the **chancre** heals, if effective treatment was not received. Because of the diversity of symptoms **syphilis** is sometimes called the great imitator. The symptoms of the secondary stage of **syphilis** usually last three to six months but can come and go periodically. After all symptoms disappear. 50 to 70 per cent of people with untreated syphilis stay in this stage for the rest of their lives."[352]

Remainder passes on to the tertiary stage or late **syphilis** which involves serious heart problem, eye problems, brain and spinal cord damage. These complications cause blindness, paralysis, death and other disabling conditions. Such developments may take up to 20 to 30 years.

For such a prolonged period, it could not have been possible to observe patients to know fate of Homeopathic treatment, so Hahnemann wrongly concluded that he had cured **syphilitic** patients by Homeopathy, same mistake was done by Kent.

Kent writes—

"Homeopathic treatment strikes at the root of the evil and painful chancre will become painless. Suppressed manifestations must come back and they will come back under appropriate treatment."[353]

Chancre of syphilis are painless already. There is no question of Homeopathic treatment which can make **syphilitic chancre** painless. It was wrong observation by Kent. Kent writes that suppressed manifestation must come back under treatment. It was also a wrong comment of Kent. Normally the first stage of **syphilis** is spontaneously suppressed. Then, after some time, secondary stage appears which is also suppressed spontaneously and after gap of years third stage appears. "The symptoms of the secondary stage of **syphilis** usually last three to six months but can come and go periodically."[354]

This periodicity of appearance and disappearance of **symptomatology** of **syphilis** gave wrong impression to Kent that reappearance of **symptomatology** of **syphilis** was due to Homeopathic treatment. But it was not the fact. Periodicity of **symptomatology** in **syphilis** and in 70 to 80 per cent of patients total disappearance of symptoms after second stage without any treatment is the normal course of **syphilis**. By above discussion we can say that the comment of Kent —"Suppressed manifestations must come back under appropriate treatment" is wrong.

Regarding frequency of doses Hahnemann writes—"A single one of which sufficiently attenuated and potentized, would have sufficed to cure all the disease in the whole habitable world for which this drug is the suitable remedy."[355] I am giving an example of *arsenicum album*. Regarding dose of *arsenic*, Hahnemann says, "Homeopathy which by unwearied, multiplied experiments discovered that it is only rare cases that more than a decillionth of a grain of arsenic should be given."[356]

One decillionth dilution means $1:10^{60}$ dilution. Hahnemann, Kent and we all agree that in such dilutions it is very difficult to find a single molecule of a drug. Example of **syphilis** is being given, where causative organism of **syphilis** is Trepanoma pallidum. How can **Trepanoma pallidum** be killed by drug which contains not even a single molecule of drug.

Hahnemann said that best Homeopathic drug should be given in single dose only with 10^{60} dilution. How can a drug kill treponema pallidum or other organism in a single dose with 10^{60} dilution. Hahnemann used *arsenic* for treatment of **syphilis** in single dose. How can *arsenic* in one globule which contains 10^{60} dilution be effective in treatment of **syphilis**.

To understand importance of dose in treatment, example of *penicillin* must be learnt.

Penicillin is the drug of choice in treatment of **syphilis**. **Trepanoma** is highly susceptible to *penicillin*. "To be effective in **syphilis** and other trepanomatoses, high blood concentration of *penicillin* 0.03 units per ml. must be attained. Moreover, because *penicillin* only attacks actively dividing organisms and trepanomas divide only slowly, this high concentration must be maintained for periods up to 15 days to ensure that all the organisms have been killed and to prevent relapses. In **syphilis** penicillin is best given in daily intramuscular doses of 600000 to one million units of *procaine penicillin G*."[357]

Neoarsphenamine, an arsenic compound, had been used in **syphilis** previously. "**Neoarsphenamine** 0.6 gm is made into solution with sterile distilled water 6 ml and the freshly made solution is injected intravenously once a week for 10 weeks."[358]

Arsenic compounds are not used today due to toxicity. But if we use arsenic then required doses have to be administered in treatment of **syphilis** to kill **Trepanoma pallidum**. The dilutions of **arsenic** used by Hahnemann cannot kill the syphilitic micro-organism. When Homeopathy does not accept Treponema pallidum as a causative organism of **syphilis**, then the question of killing treponema cannot be raised in Homeopathy. This truth should be accepted by Homeopathy that causative organism of **syphilis** is **trepanoma pallidum**, because in the absence of **trepanoma**, **syphilis** cannot be produced in human being.

Now conclusively we can say, in **syphilis** after the secondary stage, it is more or less impossible to say on the basis of healed symptoms only that disease has been cured by drug or it has been cured spontaneously or disease is in remission phase. Because this disease may remain **symptomless** up to 20 to 30 years. Observation up to 20 to 30 years, after disappearance of symptom of secondary stage of **syphilis**, is required to know that disease has been cured spontaneously or diseased state is present. Development of **neurosyphilis**, **cardiovascular syphilis** or other symptoms, which develop only after a prolonged interval are only symptomatological evidence of late **syphilis**. After secondary stage **syphilis** may remain silent for years. It is very difficult to say which patient will develop late **syphilis** and which patient will get cured spontaneously. As we know, only 17-20 per cent of **syphilitic** patients develop late symptoms of **syphilis**, remaining patients are cured spontaneously.

Hahnemann did not know about **syphilis**. So he made a wrong judgement regarding its cure. He wrongly presumed that he had been able to cure **syphilis** by Homeopathic medicine. Then he made an erroneous concept of Homeopathy.

As we know, "The average interval from infection to onset of symptoms is 5 to 10 years for **meningovascular syphilis**, 20 years for **tabes dorsalis**." These varieties of **syphilis** which develop after prolonged interval usually do not have skin lesions. These varieties of

syphilis develop after remission of secondary stage of **syphilis**. Without serological test, it is very difficult to tell that these varieties are **sequalae** of primary **syphilis** or independent of **syphilis**. At the time of Hahnemann serological test of **syphilis** was not available, that's why he was not able to detect **syphilis** in those patients who had neurological or cardiovascular complications. "Even in 1875 William Welch's report that syphilis was a cause of aortic aneurysm was ignored until 30 years later, Reuter demonstrated spirochetes within the vessel walls in active aortitis."[359]

Thus Hahnemann must have wrongly interpreted about cure of **syphilitic** patients and developed wrong concept regarding treatment of **syphilis**. Misinterpretation of treatment of **syphilis** is the most important cause in development of Homeopathy.

In the description of **syphilis**, Kent writes—"Dissimilar repel each other and similar attract and cure each other."[360]

But what is the fact—

"Untreated **syphilis** may make people more susceptible to other diseases or individuals who get **syphilis** coincidentally may be more susceptible to other diseases."[361]

Kent also writes about the Homeopathic treatment of **syphilis**—

"Homeopathic treatment strikes at the root of the evil... . bubo will be hastened to suppuration when it would not otherwise suppurate."[362]

But the fact is that "The **chancre** of primary **syphilis** is **indurated** and the associated adenopathy is bilateral, non-tender and non-suppurative."[363]

In this way we can conclude that these people of Homeopathy did not have proper knowledge of diseases that's why they erroneously diagnosed the disease. They were not able to differentiate one disease from another due to lack of knowledge.

41

*S**ycosis***, the **condylomatous** disease is ineradicable by the vital force without proper medicinal treatment. **Sycosis** is revealed by cauliflower-like growth. When discharge of **gonorrhoea** is suppressed by Allopathic injection, **sycosis** is established in the body.

ARGUMENT

We have discussed **syphilis** in detail and reached a conclusion that Hahnemann and Kent were wrong and they made wrong impressions about treatment of **syphilis**.

Now we shall discuss **sycosis**, second chronic miasm and we will be able to prove that Hahnemann was again wrong in the study of **sycosis**.

Hahnemann writes—

"According to all investigations only three chronic miasms are found. The diseases caused by which manifest themselves through local symptoms and from which most if not all the chronic diseases originate; namely first **syphilis** which I have also called the **venereal chancre disease**, then **sycosis** or the **figwart disease** and finally the chronic disease which lies at the foundation of the eruption of itch *i.e.* the **psora**."[364] All chronic diseases never pass away of themselves but increase and are aggravated even till death."[365]

"**Syphilis** and **sycosis** were called as two venereal diseases."[366] Hahnemann also writes—

"**Syphilis** and **sycosis** both have an advantage over the **itch disease** in this that the **chancre** or bubo in the one and **figwart** in the other never leave the external parts until they have been either mischievously destroyed through external repressiveremedies or have been in a rational manner removed through the simultaneous internal cure of the whole disease. The venereal disease cannot therefore break out so long as the chancre is not artificially destroyed by external applications, nor can the secondary ailments of **sycosis** break out so long as the **figwart** has not been destroyed by faulty practice, for these local symptoms which act as substitute for the internal disease, remain standing even until the end of man's life and prevent the breaking out of internal disease."[367]

Hahnemann writes regarding treatment of **syphilis** and **sycosis**—

"It is therefore just as easy to heal them even in their whole extent *i.e.* thoroughly through their specific internal medicines which need only to be continued until these local symptoms (**chancre** and **figwart**) which are in their nature unchangeable exceptthrough artificial external applications are thoroughly healed. Then we may be quite certain that we have thoroughly cured the internal disease *i.e.* syphilis and sycosis."[368]

Hahnemann writes in *Organon* of *Medicine*—

"**Sycosis** the **condylomatous** disease equally ineradicable by the vital force without proper medicinal treatment. **Sycosis** is revealed by cauliflower- like growth."[369]

Some Homeopaths explained—"Any type of muscular growth which is abnormal is actually **sycosis.** Sometimes warts like cauliflower or like a bunch of grapes are also due to **sycosis**. **External piles** are also labelled due to **sycosis**."[370]

It is written in Homeopathy that "**Gonorrhoea** is due to sexual relation with diseased females and when discharge of **gonorrhoea** is suppressed by injections of Allopathic doctors, **sycosis** is established in the body."[371]

42

Hahnemann included all venereal diseases into two groups. One where lesion is ulcerative or *papular* labelled as **syphilitic *miasm*** and second where lesion is like external growth or discharge from urethra labelled as **sycosis**. Both were called as two venereal diseases which were treated with the mercury,*thuja* and nitric acid by Hahnemann.

ARGUMENT

Today we know that there are five common venereal diseases also known as sexually transmitted diseases. These are **syphilis, gonorrhoea**, **chancroid, lymphogranuloma venereum** and **granuloma inguinale**. One more which we shall include in our discussion is **genital wart** or **condyloma acuminata**. And next **genital herpes** is important for analytical aspect of Homeopathy.

We shall discuss these seven diseases because all these spread by coitus.

To differentiate all these diseases from each other is not easy by only clinical inspection. "Early **granuloma inguinal** may be mistaken for the **primary chancre** or **condyloma latum** of **syphilis**. Chronic ulcerative or **cicatrical** changes may resemble **lymphogranuloma venereum. Amoebiasis** can produce penile lesions resembling **donovanosis (Granuloma inguinal**)."[372]

Isolation of infective agent which may be bacteria, virus, **chlamydia** or other agent and serological tests are only two confirmatory process to make a definite diagnosis. Both these methods were not present at the time of Hahnemann. Hahnemann and his followers must not have been able to make accurate diagnosis. They were confused and not able to differentiate one disease from another.

Second most important aspect is regarding treatment. Hahnemann thought—"These all above mentioned sexually transmitted diseases are due to chronic miasm and cannot be cured spontaneously." But the fact is that maximum number of patients of above sexual transmitted diseases are cured spontaneously. Diseases only in few patients become complicated or may be fatal. Death due to these sexually transmitted diseases are very few in numbers. These facts were not known to Hahnemann. He thought wrongly that he had been curing **syphilis** and **sycosis** by *mercury*, *thuja* and *nitric acid*. When he was not able to cure some patients, he said it was due to **psora** which complicated **syphilis** and **sycosis.** I have said many times that the dilutions used by Hahnemann had no drug. Such Homeopathic drugs are actually no drug. Homeopathic treatment is actually no treatment.

Hahnemann writes—

"These excrescences usually first manifest themselves on the genitals and appears usually but not always attended with a sort of **gonorrhoea** from the urethra several days or several weeks, even many weeks after infection through coition, more rarely they appear dry and like **warts** more frequently soft and spongy, emitting a specifically fetid fluid, bleeding easily and in the form of a coxcomb or a cauliflower. Usually in **gonorrhoea** of this kind the discharge is from the beginning **thickish** like pus, body of penis swollen somewhat hard and very painful to touch and in some cases covered on the back with glandular tubercles."[373]

Actually in **gonorrhoea,** there is no excrescence and no external growth. The main symptom of **gonorrhoea** is purulent discharge through urethra. Excrescence or external growth at **anogenital** region occurs in (1) **Granuloma inguinale**, (2) **Lymphogranuloma venereum**, (3) **Condylomata**, (4) **Condyloma acuminata**.

Growth in anogenital region also occurs in other conditions like carcinoma but these are non-venereal diseases. These diseases will not be discussed here because these are non-venereal and Hahnemann described only venereal disease in relation to **sycosis.** There is complete possibility that Hahnemann may have included non-venereal diseases (like carcinoma, piles etc. having external growth atanogenital region) in **sycosis** by erroneously presuming that these diseases spread by a coitus, as "mentioned by some Homeopaths."[374]

In summary we can say Hahnemann included all venereal diseases into two groups, one where lesion is ulcerative or **papular** labelled as **syphilitic miasm** and second where lesion is like an external growth or discharge from urethra, labelled as **sycosis miasm**. "Disease like **granuloma inguinale** begins as a papule which ulcerates and develops into a painless elevated zone may be mistaken for the primary chancre or **condyloma latum** of syphilis and when epithelial proliferation, resembling carcinoma in the genital or **perianal** region in a young subject should always raise the suspicion of **granuloma** inguinale."[375]

In **granuloma inguinale**—

"Less common complications of the disease include deep ulceration, chronic cicatrical lesions, phimosis, lymphedema and exuberant epithelial proliferation whichgrossly resemble carcinoma."[376]

This is my opinion that when diseases have such complications where external growth is a feature, Hahnemann must have included these in **sycosis**.

There is no necessity to differentiate diseases into **syphilis** or **sycosis**. Our intention is to prove that diseases either part of **syphilis** or **sycosis** usually resolve spontaneously and gave a wrong message to Hahnemann and Kent, and other followers that they had been curing the disease by drugs having decillionth potency.

- **Granuloma inguinal** which I have described already, develops due to bacteria known as **Calymmatobacterium granulomatis**. "Healing may occur at any stage or slow or rapid extension may continue intermittently and irregularly for years... . Temporary remissions may be followed by recrudescence which mayoccur in healed scars. When the lesions are extensive **cachexia** may occur after a weary course of many years predispose to death from **intercurrent** infection."[377] "Diagnosis depends upon the finding of the Donovan bodies in scrapping or by the biopsy. It is important to exclude **syphilis** both by dark field and by the serological examination. The lesions of **granuloma inguinal** in untreated cases after many months, tend to heal by themselves. When healing takes place, the scar may be **atrophic** and **hypopigmented** or **hypertrophic.** Some cases have been reported to develop malignancy."[378]

- The next disease, **lymphogranuloma-venereum** is a sexually transmitted infection caused by **chlamydia trachomatis.** It is characterized by "infection of lymph channels and lymph nodes manifesting by bubo formation, ulcerations, enlargement of genital organs and rectal stricture. Fever, chills, headache and joint pains may also be present. Abscess formation with drainage of pus from the inguinal lymph nodes is usual. Later manifestations of disease include secondary ulceration and elephantiasis of genitals in both sexes, polypoid growths about the anus, and inflammation, ulceration and stricture of rectum."[379] The most reliable method of diagnosis is isolation of chlamydia from aspirated bubo pus and by **immuno-diagnostic tests**. "Spontaneous healing usually occurs after several months leaving inguinal scars or granulomatous masses of varying size which persist for life."[380] "The untreated disease usually runs an average course of six to eight weeks and may then resolve completely. Many cases are left with the sequelae of lymphatic obstruction and some show periodic recrudescences of activity for many years."[381] Clinically it is difficult to distinguish this disease from **granuloma inguinal**, and **genital tuberculosis**.
- **Chancroid** (soft chancre) is an acute, specific, localized, self-limiting, **autoinoculable** infectious disease almost always acquired through sexual contact, initiated by "an infectious agent known as the Ducrey bacillus (a bacterium). It is characterized by painful ulceration at the site of inoculation usually on genitals and may be accompanied by purulent lymphadenitis."[382] "Disease of **chancroid** is self-limited and systemic spread does not occur. Without treatment genital ulcers and inguinal abscess have occasionally been reported to persist for years. Local pain is the most frequent complaint."[383]
- "**Condyloma acuminata** or **genital warts** are usually asymptomatic. Small lesions appear as 1 to 2 mm white **macules** or papules. In most cases genital warts are numerous and appear in clusters. However, solitary lesions may occur. Grape-like or cauliflower-like clustering does occur specially perennially."[384]
- This disease for diagnosis has to be differentiated from **condylomalata, carcinomas, lichen planus**, **moles, seborrheic keratoses, cyst**. It is a virus infection known as Human **papilloma** virus. More than 60 type of H.P.V. have been detected. "This virus infects the most epithelium of the **anogenital** region and results in spectrum of lesions ranging from **condyloma acuminata**, **intraepithelial neoplasia,** and **invasive squamous** cell carcinoma."[385]

- Study of **warts** is important because **sycosis miasm** includes mainly **warts** and clinically similar diseases. "**Warts** are benign neoplasm of the skin. **Warts** are found in approximately 7 to 20 per cent of the population, with the highest frequency in the early teenage years. Person to person transmission by direct contact with **wart** tissue and indirectly by virus contamination through contaminated secretions or instruments may occur. Autoinoculation of virus to contiguous or distant sites is frequent. **Warts** are skin coloured, can be single or occur in multiple clusters and are often widely dispersed over the body. **Warts** may persist and spread within the same person for several years or may recur in an individual several years after a total remission. Most studies indicate that one-third of **warts** are gone by six months and two-thirds of **warts** will resolve spontaneously within a two year period.
- During pregnancy **warts** may increase in size. The development of *antiwart antibodies* has been correlated with clinical regression in patients or those with combined immuno-deficiency, **warts** may reappear. Radical therapy of **warts** should be eschewed because most **warts** will eventually spontaneously disappear without leaving any scar."[386]
- "Children with common **warts** may not require therapy. Studies of spontaneous regression of **warts** in children suggest that 2/3 will remit within two years with remaining **verrucae** continue to resolve at this rate. However new **wart** may appear...while others are regressing."[387] "Neither the patient's age nor the number of **warts** present influences the course."[388] "Duration of genital **warts** varies from a few weeks to many years."[389]
- When treatment part of **wart** is considered. "Routine treatment of every **wart** is unnecessary and undesirable. The degree of disability must be carefully weighed against the discomfort or hazards of the proposed treatment and natural history of the **wart** and its probable spontaneous cure must be constantly borne in mind."[390]

  "Most of the innumerable folk remedies for **warts** depend for their success on the tendency of **warts** to spontaneous resolution and possibly the influence of suggestion. It is widely believed that suggestion can cure **warts**. Both the probability of spontaneous cure and the possibility of influence by suggestion must be taken into account in planning and evaluating any form of treatment."[391]
- It has been mentioned correctly—"As **warts** often disappear spontaneously, any treatment which is in use at the time will gain an undeserved reputation as a **wart** cure."[392]

- It is also found that when one **wart** is treated by topical application, other **warts** present over the body disappear suddenly. In this phenomenon immunity plays an important role.
- "**Genital herpes** is a viral infection, generally transmitted by sexual contact. **Genital herpes** is marked by clusters of small painful blisters on the genitals. After a few days these blisters burst leaving small ulcers in their place. Almost all cases are marked by painful burning at the site of blister formation. Other relatively common symptoms include pain or burning during urination, discharge from the urethra or vagina and tender swollen lymph nodes in the groin, but all these tend to disappear within one or two weeks. If generalized symptoms such as headache or fever appear, they diminish gradually over first week of the infection. After the blisters burst, lesions usually heal in one to two weeks. Skin lesions last an average of 16.5 days in men and 19.7 days in women. Although the blisters disappear and the ulcers heal spontaneously within one to three weeks but many people have recurrent episodes of **genital herpes** varying in frequency from once a month to once every few years. Fortunately many who suffer from **herpes** find that repeat attacks tend to die out after a few years."[393]
- **Gonorrhoea** is a bacterial infection caused by Neisseria gonorrhoe, a gram negative coccus. **Gonorrhoea** in a male is characterized by purulent urethral discharge, dysuria and frequent urination. Other local complications are inguina lymphadenitis, edema of penis and abscess. In homosexual men anorectal and pharyngeal infections are common. In female dysuria, frequent urination, increased vaginal discharge, anorectal dyscomfort, midline low abdominal pain and tenderness are common symptoms of **gonorrhoea.** "Before antibiotic treatment became available symptoms of **urethritis** persisted for an average of eight weeks and **unilateral epididymitis** occurred in 5 to 10 per cent untreated men."[394] In homosexual men **symptomatology** of **gonorrhoea**, "may subside without treatment, leaving a chronic asymptomatic carrier state."[395]
- "Symptoms gradually resolve without treatment but it is not known how long patients remain infectious, the longer patients remain without treatment the more likely they are to develop complications."[396]
- "From one to three per cent of adults with gonococcal infection develop gonococcemia. The onset of gonococcemia is characterized by fever, polyarthralgias and papular, petechial, pustular, haemorrhagic or necrotic skin lesions. Wrists, fingers, knee and

ankles are most often involved joints. Without treatment, the duration of **gonococcemia** is variable, the systemic manifestations of **bacteremia** may subside spontaneously within a week."[397]

- **External haemorrhoids** is not a sexually transmitting disease. Some Homeopaths include this disease in **sycosis**. "A thrombosed external **haemorrhoids** appears suddenly and is very painful. The **haematoma** is usually situated in a lateralregion of the anal margin. In the majority of cases resolution or fibrosis occurs. Indeed this condition has been called a five day painful, self-curing lesion."[398]
- **Condyloma lata** are skin lesions of secondary **syphilis**. These lesions also subside spontaneously.

At the time of Hahnemann, differential diagnosis of various sexual transmitted disease was not possible. "Until the nineteenth century, genital **warts** were believed to be a form of **syphilis** and **gonorrhoea**."[399]

This mistake was made by Hahnemann and Kent. All diseases which were presumed due to **syphilis** and **sycosis** miasm usually resolved spontaneously. This gave false observation to Hahnemann and Kent that they had been curing these diseases.

As written by Hahnemann—

"The **gonorrhoea** dependent on the figwart miasm as well as the above mentioned excrescence (the whole **sycosis**) are cured most surely and most thoroughly through the internal use of **thuja** which in this case is Homeopathic in a dose of a few pellets as large as poppy seeds, moistened with the dilution potentized to the decillionth degree and when these have exhausted their action after fifteen, twenty, thirty, forty days alternating with just as small a dose of *nitric acid* diluted to the **decillionth** degree which must be allowed to act as long a time in order to remove the **gonorrhoea** and the excrescence—the whole **sycosis**."[400] In this way Hahnemann made the wrong concept of Homeopathy.

43

It had been thought previously that **syphilis** always follows on the destruction of **chancre** by local applications and Allopathic drugs modify acute diseases into chronic diseases which become very troublesome to people.

ARGUMENT

Development of knowledge is a continuous process. Even in medical science, what was acceptable in 1900, has been discarded today.

- "In 1892, Guanieri gave the first clear description of **smallpox** what he believed to be a parasitic protozoan."[401] But today we know with absolute proof that it was a virus infection. Previously, "local treatment of the **chancre**,"[402] was indicated in Allopathy which was opposed by Hahnemann but in modern medical science at present no local treatment is indicated in **syphilis** and **gonorrhoea**.

  When medical concept of 1900 is not acceptable today on the basis of new inventions and new discoveries then how can the old unscientific and hypothetical concept of Homeopathy be accepted today?

I am giving some more examples how Hahnemann made— wrong conclusions—

- Hahnemann quoted John Hunter. John Hunter says—not one patient out of fifteen will escape **syphilis** if the **chancre** is destroyed by mere external applications. Fabre declares—**syphilis** always follows on the destruction of the chancre by local applications."[403] This was the wrong conclusion. Today we know even without localized destruction of **chancre**, **syphilis** will remain and spread in the body. Appearance of secondary stage of **syphilis** is not related in anyway with the local destruction of **chancre**.

- Hahnemann writes at one place —"I have never, in my practice of more than 50 years seen any trace of the venereal disease break out so long as the **chancre** remained untouched in its place even if this were a space of several years."[404]

  It was actually **chancroid** not **chancre**, which has been wrongly understood **chancre** by Hahnemann. Because "during medieval time **chancroid** was not distinguished from the initial lesion of **syphilis** but it was not until 1850 that soft **chancre** was distinguished from the initial lesion of **syphilis** and later designated **chancroid** (**chancre** like)."[405]

  In some cases of **chancroid** "untreated **chancroid** ulcers persist for long periods of time and often progress."[406]

- Hahnemann also said at various places that "Allopathic drugs modified acute diseases into chronic diseases."[407] and "Chronic diseases which are produced by Allopathy are very troublesome to people."[408] "Chronic medical **dyscrasia** so often produced by Allopathic bungling along with the natural disease left uncured by it require a much longer time for their recovery often indeed, are they incurable."[409] Hahnemann also mentioned that allopathic drugs when removed external manifestations or discharge, disease redirected internally from surface and creates various systemic symptoms. Hahnemann repeatedly mentioned that Allopathic drugs are very dangerous. Hahnemann was right because during his time antibiotics had not been discovered. Metals and its compounds were used in various diseases and these compounds were very toxic that's why they are not used today.

In spontaneously curable diseases Allopathic drugs developed various toxic manifestations while Homeopathic drugs were totally harmless. Homeopathic drugs have no effect and no side effect. Spontaneously curable diseases will be cured without help of any drug. By the help of Homeopathic drugs,Hahnemann protected the population from toxic manifestations of old Allopathic procedures.

44

Allopathic drugs suppress symptoms to redirect them internally and create various systemic disturbances. By suppression of **psora**, **syphilis** and **sycosis** after administration of Allopathic Injections, many types of disease symptoms are produced.

ARGUMENT

Hahnemann had one more typical argument about suppression of external symptoms.

Hahnemann was of the opinion that all external symptoms and externally localized lesions are part of internal diseases. Hahnemann said, "When external symptoms or externally localized lesions are removed by internally used Homeopathic drug then it is alright. But when externally localized lesions or symptoms are removed by internally used Allopathic drugs, it is wrong." He said, "When allopathic drugs are used, they suppress symptoms then disease redirected internally and create various disorders."

Hahnemann thought, that Homeopathic drugs cure symptoms while Allopathic drugs suppress symptoms and create systemic disturbances. How did Hahnemann reach such a conclusion? Homeopathic drugs actually do not cure the disease and never produce side effect while Allopathic drugs used in the sexually transmitted disease at the time of Hahnemann were very toxic irrespective of the therapeutic effect. "Many chemicals are toxic to cell protoplasm. Effect upon cells may be non-selective and cells of the host as well as invading bacteria may be killed."[410]

Mercuric metallic ion gets absorbed on the surface of bacterium and then enters and coagulates the protoplasm. *Mercury* like *arsenic* combines with sulphhydril groups in the bacterial cell thus interfering with cellular metabolism."[411] "*Mercury* while not being an active **spirochaeticide** accumulates in the **syphilitic** lesions and inhibit the development of organism. But coincidental with such a **spirochaetostatic** effect appear symptoms of chronic mercurialism.*Bismuth* took the place of *mercury* until the development of *penicillin* treatment."[412] In the preantibiotic era, "*Antimony* compounds were the standby in the treatment of the disease—**granuloma venereum**."[413]

"Results with *mercury* treatment in **syphilis** were far from satisfactory for the attendant**mercurialism** coupled with doubtful result within a few decades of its birth, arsenic treatment has become obsolete in **syphilis**. Toxic complications during the necessary prolonged*arsenic* therapy often claimed as high a mortality as the disease itself. *Bismuth* introduced in 1922 as a substitute for*mercury* as complement to *arsenic*, served purpose to some extent. *Penicillin* today has been proved to be curative in **syphilis** beyond any claim of the earlier drugs."[414] "Bismuth immobilized the spirochetes (causative organism of **syphilis**) rendering them non-infectious. *Bismuth* may, therefore, be stated to prevent the spread and multiplication of spirochetes and depress the disease to a point where the degree of resistance already existing in the body can control the infection."[415] "Unlike the organic *arsenicals* which have fallen out in complete disuse in the therapy of **syphilis**, *bismuth* and its compounds are still in use as an adjunct to *penicillin* therapy in *latent* **syphilis** and **cardiovascular syphilis**."[416]

"*Antimony* and *potassium tartrate* was first used in the treatment of **granuloma inguinale**. The injections are given at intervals of two to three days, 10 to 12 injections may clear the lesions sufficiently."[417]

In Allopathy, chemicals were used in the treatment of various sexually transmitted diseases at the time of Hahnemann. We also know that differential diagnosis was also not clear at that time. **Syphilis** may have been diagnosed as **gonorrhoea** and **chancroid** may have been diagnosed as **chancre**. Now we also know this fact that these chemicals were used in sexually transmitted diseases in high concentration repeatedly in the form of injections and these are highly toxic. We have observed in reference no. 414 that toxic complications during the necessary prolonged *arsenic* therapy often claimed as high a mortality as the disease itself. And in reference no. 412, we understand that **spirochaeticidal** concentration of *mercury* produces symptoms of *chronic* **mercurialism**. Hahnemann said that Allopathic drugs suppressed the disease, which produced various internal ailments.

Homeopath says—

"By suppression of **psora, syphilis** and **sycosis** after administration of Allopathic injections many types of disease symptoms are produced. Gradually liver, spleen and other abdominal organs are damaged. Abdominal problems are seen. Tubercular and other chronic problems are also developed due to this suppression."[418]

By the above discussion it is clear that administration of Allopathic drugs does not produce new disease symptoms by suppressing external manifestations. Allopathic drugs cured some sexually transmitted diseases at the time of Hahnemann but produced many toxic symptoms. These toxic symptoms were misunderstood by Hahnemann as a new disease. New disease of different aetiology cannot be produced by Allopathic drugs. How can tubercular disease, caused by a bacteria be developed by Allopathic drug.

45

Figwart disease is the result of suppression of **gonorrhoea** by Allopathic treatment. Suppression of symptoms increase severity of disease. Kent concluded that Allopathic drugs suppressed **gonorrhoea** in male and after marriage this suppressed **gonorrhoea** *is* transmitted to female and causes many symptoms.

ARGUMENT

"Kent said that there are two types of **gonorrhoea**, one is acute having a tendency to recover after a few weeks or months. The acute may really and truly be called a **gonorrhoea** because all there is of it is this discharge. The suppression of acute **gonorrhoea** cannot bring on the constitutional symptoms called **sycosis**. Figwarts and constitutional symptoms will follow suppression of the chronic **miasm** and become very serious. Most of the cases of true **sycosis** that are brought before the physician at the present time are those that have been suppressed."[419]

Kent said that **Figwart disease** is the result of suppression of **gonorrhoea** by Allopathic treatment. It is absolutely wrong. **Figwart disease** is a viral infection and **gonorrhoea** is a bacterial infection, both diseases are different. It is not possible that suppression of **gonorrhoea** results in **Figwart disease**. This is entirely different matter that both diseases can exist together. Surprisingly it has been found by observations that other venereal diseases and **Figwart Disease** usually coexist together.

"In the past, **genital warts** were termed as **gonorrhoeal** or **venereal warts**. These terms are misleading and should not be used, although such patients quite often have associated venereal disease."[420]

This coexistence of both diseases confused Hahnemann and Kent who made a false statement that suppression of **gonorrhoea** (venereal disease) produces **Figwart disease**.

Suppression of symptoms may mask the disease and may give a false impression that the disease has been cured. Kent and Hahnemann repeatedly said that suppression of symptoms increase severity of disease and after that internal organs are affected. It is not correct.

Collection of pus, rotten tissue, abnormal growth, stone in important organs haveto be removed from the body and such removal is not a part of only symptomatic improvement, it is actual cure. Removal of pain and fever only are parts of symptomaticimprovement. We should not confuse about these two concepts.

Kent said that if a female suffered from "In a year or eighteen months after marriage with uterine trouble, with ovarian disease, with abdominal troubles, with all sorts of complaints peculiar to the woman and it has been found that her husband had two three attacks of **gonorrhoea** that were treated with Allopathic drugs."[421]

Kent concluded that Allopathic drugs suppressed **gonorrhoea** in male and after marriage this suppressed **gonorrhoea** transmitted to female and caused many mentioned symptoms. "Kent also said suppression of **gonorrhoea** leads to **anaemia**."[422]

Kent said symptoms mentioned in reference no.421 and reference 422 are due to suppressed **gonorrhoea**. It was only imagination and hypothesis of Kent. There are hundreds of causes of these symptoms. Without isolation of bacteria and serological test, nothing can be said. In **gonorrhoea** we know that "acute symptoms of gonococcal**urethritis** in the female may subside spontaneously."[423]

"Symptoms gradually resolve without treatment but it is not known how long patients remain infectious."[424] That's why without confirming diagnosis of disease such type of hypothesis should not be accepted. At the time of Hahnemann and Kent there were confusions in diagnosis of disease. This confusion and wrong diagnosis created misnomer and wrong hypothesis which are being accepted by Homeopaths and their followers, *e.g.* "until the nineteenth century **genital warts** were believed to be a form of **syphilis** or **gonorrhoea.**"[425] Such wrong concepts are mainly responsible for origin of Homeopathy.

In reference no. 421, it should be clear in the mind of readers that suppression of **gonorrhoea** was mentioned in male and after one year from suppression his wife suffered from many symptoms which Kent said due to **gonorrhoea,** transmitted from husband. Here I say that **symptomatology** in the female was definitely due to something other than **gonorrhoea** because at that time no accurate diagnostic facilities were available and there were no knowledge about other diseases of females. We also know today that "in most cases of **gonorrhoea** there are few systemic symptoms beyond malaise and a slight headache."[426] How can all gynaecological problems of females be correlated with **gonorrhoea**. Such correlation is unscientific and baseless.

Kent described many symptoms due to suppression of **gonorrhoea.** Kent said—"Sometimes it is so severe in form and the trouble comes so soon after the suppression that there can be no doubt even in the mind of the man himself, that the trouble he is now suffering from relates to the suppression of that discharge. Sometimesthey are latent and develop very gradually and the blood becomes affected andgradually increasing **anaemia** comes and the patient being pallid and waxy."[427]

According to Kent **sycosis** means suppressed **gonorrhoea** and **Figwart disease** is a **sycotic** trouble.

Kent writes—"A man who has gone from 10 to 15 years with this **sycotic** trouble. He is waxy, subject to various kinds of figwarts, his lips are pale and his ears almost transparent, he has various kinds of manifestations that we call symptoms. Thetrouble may have manifested itself in other mucous membranes of the body and thus saved the man from his waxiness. He is not so pallid when the condition becomes busy in another region. These catarrhal manifestations may be catarrhal conditions of the eyes but are commonly catarrhs of the nose. It is not an uncommon thing for a nasal catarrh to be **sycotic** and to have existed only since the **gonorrhoea** was suppressed. The catarrh is located in the nose and posterior nares with thick copious discharge."[428]

Kent further explained that suppression of **gonorrhoeal** discharge creates internal pathology and gives rise to many symptoms. When treatment has been done by Homeopathic drug, suppressed **gonorrhoeal** discharge should be brought externally from the nose. "When the constitution is vigorous enough it will keep up the discharge inspite of the different specific remedies that have been administered but in constitutions that are feeble, diseases are easily driven to the centre, leaving the outermost parts of man."[429]

In this way what Homeopathy says is that discharge should come back externally. Kent writes—"So it is often the case that a man with a thick yellowish-green discharge from the nose after a dose of *calcarea* which is an antisycotic, one of the deepest in character, has his old discharge, brought back."[430]

Kent also said – "If the catarrh does not come on soon the constitution is too weak for the catarrh to represent the disease and it will be represented on deeper tissues. **Bright's disease** may come, breaking down of the lungs, breaking down of the liver, rheumatic affection of the worst form finally killing the patient."[431]

Kent said that if **gonorrhoeal** discharge does not come out of the body in catarrhal form, it will damage many internal organs in male and female. Kent writes – "Sometimes in the man it does not take the catarrhal form but produces inflammation of the testes or it may affect the rectum. Again if you go to the bedside of a man who has used strong injections for the purpose of suppressing a **gonorrhoeal** discharge and you find him in bed writhing and turning, tossing, twisting with the pain and the only relief for him is to keep in continual motion, the pains are tremendous, they are rending and tearing from head to foot."[432]

Kent and Hahnemann both said that suppression of **gonorrhoeal** discharge is responsible for creating many new signs and symptoms of internal pathology. And I say it was wrong observation of Hahnemann and Kent. The signs and symptoms of internal pathology were due to toxicity of Allopathic drugs given for treatment of sexually atransmitted disease.

I have written previously that at the time of Hahnemann compounds of *mercury*, *arsenic* and *bismuth* were used as chemotherapeutic agents. The standard method of treatment was "to administer a variable number of *neoarsphenamine* and to supplement these with intramuscular injections of mercury or bismuth. The whole treatment extends over a period of two years."[433]

"Regular administration of *arsenic* in any soluble form does not produce tolerance but on the contrary produces cumulative poisoning. The *arsenic* retained is distributed throughout the body."[434]

"*Mercury* was the first drug to be used as a specific disinfectant. Satisfactory results are only produced by *mercury* after prolonged action and the minimum efficient therapeutic concentration of *mercury* closely approaches the toxic concentration. *Mercury* is excreted very slowly and hence has a marked cumulative action. This metal was stored in various organs and particularly in the kidney and liver. After a course of mercurial treatment, the body gets rid of the *mercury* very slowly and small quantities continue to be excreted for three months after the last dose has been given."[435]

Administration of these metallic compounds may have cured the diseases or diseases were cured spontaneously but this is certain that these drugs must have produced many symptoms due to toxicity which Hahnemann and Kent said originated dueto suppression of **gonorrhoea**. Some toxicity of these metallic compounds appeared onthe surfacc like increased discharge through mouth and nose that has been called by Hahnemann and Kent as reappearance of discharge through mouth and nose as written in reference no. 394. "Salivation and *gingivitis* are the first symptoms of **mercurial poisoning**. The salivation is often very marked and several litres of saliva may be secreted a day."[436] Hahnemann has written that "*mercury* has been used internally."[437]

"The mucous membranes of the throat, nose become inflamed with an associated **conjunctivitis** in **chronic arsenic poisoning**."[438] "Iodine and its salts are the second remedy for **syphilis**. Abundant nasal discharge, swelling of the nasal and ocular fever, headache and general malaise may form a true **iodic influenza**."[439] Kent emphasized that nasal catarrh and catarrh of other mucous membrane are due to suppression of **gonorrhoea** but now we can say it is due to toxicity of drugs used by Allopathic doctors.

Arsenic which was used by Allopathic doctors also causes "perspiration, excessive salivation, sweating, stomatitis, sore throat, **coryza**, lacrimation"[440] and such type of action of Allopathic drugs confused Hahnemann and Kent who said these are symptoms of suppressed **gonorrhoea** which comes out externally by Homeopathic drugs. At the time of Hahnemann there was no knowledge about toxicity of these metallic compounds and there were no pharmacokinetic and pharmacodynamic studies of these compounds. As mentioned rightly: "There have been epidemics of **mercury poisoning** among wildlife and human populations in many countries. With very few exceptions and for numerous reason such outbreaks were misdiagnosed for months or even years. Factors in these tragic delays included the insidious onset of the **affliction**, vagueness of early clinical signs and the medical profession's unfamiliarity with the disease."[441]

Kent writes—"It is often the case that a man with a thick yellowish-green discharge from the nose after a dose of calcarea, which is an **antisycotic**, one of the deepest in character has his old discharge brought back."[442] We know from the knowledge of chemistry that many compounds of *mercury* and *arsenic* are coloured. “In **arsenic poisoning** there is high coloured, bloody stool.”[443] “In **chronic arsenic poisoning** gums become red and soft and the tongue is coated with a thin white silvery fur.”[444] **“Gingivitis** due to mercury poisoning may be due to mercury lining precipitated in the gums as mercury sulphide by the sulphurated hydrogen present in the mouth.”[445]

“Mercuric sulphide is obtained as a black precipitate, turns red on sublimation and gradually also turns red and crystalline.”[446]

Kent observed coloured nasal discharge after Homeopathic drug administration and said that the old discharge is being brought back. It was wrong. Actually, it was toxicity of metallic compounds, Administered by Allopathic doctors.

Kent described manifestations of suppressed **gonorrhoea** as “patient being pallid and waxy, anemia comes, patient has various kinds of manifestation, catarrh conditions of the eyes and nose, breaking down of the lungs, breaking down of the liver, **Bright's disease** may come, rheumatic affection of the worst form finally killing the patient and he becomes anaemic, tremendous pain, tendons will begin to contract and they will shorten the muscles of the calves, the muscles of the thighs will become so sore that they cannot be touched or handled, sometimes there is infiltration of the muscles and hardness and this soreness extends to the bottom of the feet so that it is impossible forthe patient to walk.”[447]

These manifestations which were described by Kent due to suppression of **gonorrhoea** were in fact manifestations of chronic toxicity of metallic compound used for Allopathic treatment, as described below:

“Abdominal pain, dry and congested throat symptoms of **neuritis** are more pronounced severe cramps in the muscles which are extremely tender on pressure, patient is very restless and cannot sleep and there may be death. In cases which end in recovery, **chronic peripheral neuritis** may persist. These are sub-acute toxicity of *arsenic*. Chronic toxicity of arsenic has the following features: malaise, salivation, colicky pain, constipation, vomiting of glary mucous tinged with bile, gums are red soft, cough with expectoration, liver and kidney are damaged, **epithelioma** may develop in 20 per cent of these cases, tingling and numbness of the extremities, hyperasthesia of the skin, marked tenderness and cramps of the muscles **arthralgia** and circumscribed oedema, **aplastic anaemia**, **peripheral neuritis**, muscular atrophy, etc.”[448]

“Compounds of *mercury* when taken internally for a prolonged period, symptoms begin to appear. These are nausea, digestive disturbances, colicky pain, vomiting, **diarrhoea,** salivation is a constant symptom, swollen and painful salivary glands, inflamed and ulcerated gums which occasionally present a brownish-blue line at their junction with teeth and rarely necrosis of the jaw develops, *brownish* deposit of **mercury** on the anterior lens capsule, peripheral **neuritis**, **anaemia** and kidney damage, **mental depression**, loss of memory, insomnia, delusions and hallucinations."[449]

"Sazerac and Lavaditi (1922) showed that *bismuth* was a powerful spirochaeticide, the drug rapidly attained popularity as a substitute for mercury in the treatment of **syphilis**. *Bismuth* salts when used in the treatment of **syphilis** are always given intramuscularly. The toxic actions produced by *bismuth* are very similar to those produced by *mercury*. Blue gum line and salivation also occur. More serious effects aremalaise, and loss of weight, **diarrhoea**, **albuminuria**, **dermatitis** and jaundice."[450]

Now we know that symptoms of suppressed **gonorrhoea** are the same as toxic symptoms produced by metallic compounds used in sexually transmitted diseases. There is nothing like suppression of disease by Allopathic drug. It is also wrong that Homeopathic drugs bring back the manifestation of disease.

Either diseases had been cured spontaneously or diseases were cured by metallic compounds. Administered metallic compounds produced toxic symptomatology for which Kent said, symptoms are coming back by Homeopathic drugs. Later on when toxic symptomatology was resolved gradually then Kent said, "This is the cure done by Homeopathy."

Actually Homeopathic drugs have no effect, no side effect, no therapeutic utility.

46

Suppressed manifestations must come back and they will come back under appropriate treatment.

ARGUMENT

Statements of Homeopathy on different subjects are interrelated. They cannot be isolated. They are interdependent also. That's why arguments against different basic concepts of Homeopathy are also interrelated. No clear-cut demarcation is possible and chances of repetition are there. So for the argument against basic concept of Homeopathy, please study argument forty-five and forty-six.

Kent writes about **syphilis** that suppressed manifestations must come back and they will come back under appropriate treatment. I have written previously that periodicity of recurrence of**syphilitic** symptoms before spontaneous cure presented false impression that suppressed manifestations are coming back. Another cause of this false opinion was toxicity of Allopathic drugs used in the treatment of sexually transmitted disease. It had been said that *mercury* and *arsenic* suppressed manifestations of **syphilis** which should come back for actual cure. For treatment of **syphilis** *arsenic* and *mercury* were given.

"*Arsenic* has a marked toxic action on the heart, liver and kidneys. If the patient survives the gastrointestinal irritation, he may die later from injury to the vital organs. In chronic poisoning, the first visible effect is a discolouration of the skin which may vary from grey to brown and keratosis occurs in the palms and soles. **Conjunctivitis** and **laryngitis** are common. Occasionally **jaundice** and **cirrhosis** are produced."[451] "Jaundice may appear a few days after the administration of an *organic arsenical* but this type of early jaundice is rarely fatal. It is uncertain to what extent jaundice occurring during treatment is due to the drug or disease. **Syphilis** can cause considerable damage to the liver and jaundice may occur in untreated cases. Occasionally jaundice develops a considerable time after the treatment has been concluded. In this case also it is uncertain whether the condition is due to drug or to the disease."[452] Toxicity of mercuric compounds and **syphilis** give more or less similar clinical manifestations, that's why it is not easy to decide that it is drug toxicity or **syphilitic** manifestations.

Frederick Forchheimer has written rightly in 1913, "A too-prolonged administration of the drug occasions, a toxic **chloroanaemia** shown by general lassitude, insomnia, loss of weight and even *cachexia* that may be readily confounded with the similar condition incident to early **syphilitic** poisoning or extensive late lesions complicated with secondary infections. The differentiation between the two is not easy to make by watching the results of treatment. Every once in a while there comes into my wards at the city hospital a patient in a deplorable general condition emaciated, bedridden covered with ulcerative gummata or with bone or **internal syphilis**. Sometimes this patient is suffering from **syphilis** and septic infection and then *mercury* and other antisyphilitic remedies act like a charm, all the symptoms improve rapidly and the drug properly administered not only cures the symptoms of active diseases but is an absolute tonic and reconstituent. But sometimes the patient has had vigorous treatment before and gets progressively worse under mercury, iodine or arsenic. Stop all internal medication for such a patient, save mild local measures, put his bed where he can have plenty of light and air, give him as much milk and most nutritious diet possible and behold improvement starts in at once and progresses rapidly. I have seen such patients with most extensive tertiary ulceration have every one healed in a month under nothing but a simple boric acid *w.e.f.* dressing and gain weight at the rate of a pound a day. They are suffering from **chronic hydrargyrism** rather than from **syphilis**."[453]

With this statement of Frederick it is very clear that suppressed manifestations of **syphilis** was due to toxic manifestations of metallic compounds. To these patients nothing should be given. Patients would be alright when toxic manifestations subside. These toxic manifestation were also labelled as suppressed manifestations are released due to Homeopathic treatment and "bringing out external manifestations upon his body somewhere,"[454] as said by Kent.

47

Psora is that most ancient, most universal most destructive disease which has become the mother of various acute and chronic non-venereal diseases. The origin of **psora** is related to spiritualism. It is a spiritual sickness. Wrong thoughts and wrong desires give origin to **psora** and it makes the person susceptible to all diseases.

ARGUMENT

Now I am analyzing an important part of Homeopathic concept. Hahnemann said, "**Psora** is that most ancient, most universal, most misapprehended chronic miasmatic disease which for many thousands of years has disfigured and tortured mankind and which during the last centuries has become the mother of all the thousands of incredibly various (acute and) chronic (non-venereal) diseases by which the whole civilized human race on the inhabitated globe is being more and more afflicted."[455]

Kent writes—"**Psora** is the beginning of all physical sickness. Had **psora** never been established as a **miasm** upon the human race, the other two chronic diseases and susceptibility to acute diseases would have been impossible. All the diseases of man are built upon **psora** hence it is the foundation of sickness. All other sickness came afterwards."[456]

According to Homeopathy, **psora** is the most important miasm and the root of all the diseases. Now the important thing is to know about the origin of **psora.** How did **psora** originate?

Kent said—"Origin of **psora** is related with spiritualism. When persons went against the religion **psora** originated. If the human race had remained in a state of perfect order **psora** could not have existed.... It is the spiritual sickness from which first state the race progressed into what may be called the true susceptibility to **psora** which in turn laid the foundation for other diseases."[457]

Kent also explained, "Thinking and willing establishes a state in man that identifies the condition he is in. As long as man continued to think that which was true and held that which was good to the neighbour, that which was upright and just, so long man remained upon the earth free from the susceptibility to disease because that was the state in which he was created. So long as he remained in that state and preserved his integrity, he was not susceptible to disease and he gave forth no aura that could cause contagion but when man began to will the things that were the outcome of his false thinking then he entered a state which was the perfect correspondence of his interior as the life of man or as the will of man so is the body of man."[458]

Kent says, "It is the wrong thought and wrong desires which give origin to **psora** and this **psora** makes him susceptible to all diseases. Environment cannot make him susceptible to diseases. Environment is not the cause of disease." "The internal state of man is prior to that which surrounds him therefore environment is not the cause, it is only as it were a sounding board. It only reacts upon and reflects the internal. One who has the prior, which is internal, may have that which can follow upon the external, it flows as it were from the internal and effects its forms upon the skin, upon the organs, upon the body of man."[459]

Hahnemann also said that **syphilis** and **sycosis** were also complicated by coexistence of **psora**. In **syphilis** and **sycosis**, lesions were externally localized but after destruction of externally localized lesions, disease spreads into internal organs due to presence of **psora**. Hahnemann writes—"**Syphilis** and **sycosis** when complicated with developed **psora,** it is impossible to cure the venereal disease alone without treating **psora**."[460]

Various concepts were made by Hahnemann and Kent regarding origin and development of **psora**. When we analyse these concepts in the context of present medical knowledge we find that conclusions drawn in Homeopathy about **psora** were also inaccurate and false.

48

God warned that he should be followed, otherwise men will suffer from **tuberculosis** and fever. During evolution *psora* was in the form of St. Anthony's fire, during middle ages it reassumed the form of **leprosy**.

ARGUMENT

Homeopathy says, "During evolution **psora** was in the form of St. Anthony's fire, during middle ages reassumed the form of **leprosy**."[461]

Hahnemann supported religion in prevention of diseases. He took support of Moses who had said, "bodily defects which must not be found in a priest who is to offer sacrifice."[462]

Kent also said, "Patient is so well-instructed not to do anything to take no drugs to keep the life as pure as possible, to keep the physical forces untrammeled by violence."[463]

Kent writes, "Hence this states the state of human mind and the state of the human body is a state of susceptibility to disease from willing evils, from thinking that which is false and making life one continuous heredity of false things, and so this form of disease, **psora** is but an outward manifestation of that which is prior in man."[464]

"**Leprosy** prevails today upon the face of the earth but it prevails in a milder form in the form of **psora.** A new contagion comes with every child. As **psora** piles up generation after generation, century after century the susceptibility to it increases."[465]

Hahnemann took the concept of origin of **psora** from the Bible. It is mentioned in the Bible that, "Whatever a man thinks, he thinks bad. God observed, evils have beenincreased on the earth. Then God decided to punish men."[466]

"God warned that he should be followed otherwise men will be suffered from **tuberculosis** and fever."[467]

Kent mentioned, "Long before the time of Noah's flood, which was an inundation that destroyed the evil ones that were upon the earth at that time, there was a manifestation called **leprosy** which was but the result of the dreadful profanity that took place in this period. A great many people suffered then from the violent aura of **leprosy** whereas the natural disorder of the human race today is a milder form of **psora** upon a different race of people. If we had the same race upon the earth today we would have **leprosy** among them as we now have the milder form of **psora**. The ancients referred to **leprosy** as an internal itch."[468]

Noah's flood is mentioned in the Bible. It has been said that "Noah was a religious person that's why he had been protected by God and other persons on earth were non-religious and full of evils therefore they all were destroyed by flood."[469] Kent said that prior to Noah's flood many people had suffered from the violent aura and **leprosy** and this leprosy was nothing but a form of **psora**. Hahnemann writes, "The occidental **psora** which during the middle ages, had raged in Europe for several centuries under the form of **malignant erysipelas** called St. Anthony's fire, reassumed the form of **lepsoy**."[470]

What is St. Anthony's fire? St. Anthony's fire was actually toxic manifestations of **ergot poisoning**. "Ergot is a fungus to which rye is particularly susceptible. The eating of bread made from contaminated rye was responsible in the past for many outbreaks of **ergotism**. The effect of **ergotism** are alarming and explained why the disease was once regarded with superstitious dread. The most usual symptoms of **ergotism** was **gangrene** which was a consequence of vasoconstriction and which resulted in fingers, toes or whole limbs becoming dried, shrivelled and black so that they sometimes fell off.... It was for this reason (and perhaps also because the blackened limbs appeared to have been charred by fire) that **ergotism** was popularly known as St. Anthony's fire. St. Anthony's name was attached because it was believed that pilgrims to his shrine would be cured of this application. This promise did not go entirely unfulfilled for the act of pilgrimage ensured that the victim left the area in which the infected rye was growing. **Ergotism** is also associated with the occurrence of spontaneous abortions and with disturbance of central nervous function including convulsions and acute mania."[471]

St. Anthony's fire was misunderstood as a punishment of non-religious act. But in fact it was toxic manifestations of ergot, a compound present in rye. This compound was not present in bread made in shrine of St. Anthony because crops of this area was not contaminated with infected rye. When people remained in shrine of St. Anthony they must not have suffered from St. Anthony's fire.

Homeopathy is one of the best example where lack of knowledge is responsible for development of wrong therapeutic method.

- First and the most important concept which is absolutely wrong is the concept of **psora**. Whatever Hahnemann said about **psora** is absolutely wrong. He said, "**Psora** originated due to wrong thought and **psora** was modified into St. Anthony's fire and **leprosy**. All diseases except **syphilis** and **sycosis** are due to **psora**."
- Conclusion derived by Hahnemann after observation of **leprosy** patients was also wrong. In **leprosy**, "various clinical forms attack superficial tissues especially the skin, peripheral nerves and nasal mucosa."[472] Rest of the body remains healthy. Hahnemann concluded, "This was owing to the obstinately persistent eruption on the skin, which served as a substitute for the internal psora."[473] Hahnemann saidpersistency of external eruption is must to maintain health. He erroneously understood in **leprosy** that external symptomatic lesions are responsible to maintain health of **leprosy** patients and he made a wrong generalization of it. Hecommitted this mistake due to lack of knowledge. "Even in the most advanced lepromatous cases destructive lesions are limited to the skin, peripheral nerves, anterior portion of the eye, upper respiratory passages above the larynx, testes structures of the hands and feet. The probable reason for the predilection of the disease for these tissues is that they are all usually several degrees cooler than 37°C. In mice that have been experimentally infected in the foot pads, bacillary multiplication is maximal when the mice are kept at air temperature at which the foot pad tissues are about 30°C and this is also the usual temperature of the most severely involved tissues of human being."[474]
- "As one studying the lesions of **leprosy** clinically, it is evident that mycobacterium **leprae**, causative organism of **leprosy**, appears to grow best in parts of the bodythat are relatively cool.'[475] In **leprosy**,

destruction of comparatively cooler parts of body is the characteristic feature. These are not the external symptoms which make the remaining body healthy. In this way, so many wrong observations and wrong generalizations were made by Hahnemann.

49

After the destruction of external skin eruptions **psora** plays the sad role of causing innumerable secondary symptoms. When skin eruptions subside severe manifestations are the result. **Psora** spreads from one person to another person. When internal development of **psora** has been completed, vital force develops skin eruption as a substitute for the internal *psora* and keeps the **psora** in confined and stable position.

ARGUMENT

Hahnemann writes about causes of chronic diseases—"At the end of the fifteenth century, **psora** appeared only in the form of the common eruption of itch."[476] "In the last three centuries of its chief symptom (the external skin eruption) **psora** plays the sad role of causing innumerable secondary symptoms."[477] "The **psora** which is now so easily and so rashly robbed of its ameliorating cutaneous symptom the eruption of itch, which acts vicariously for the internal disease has been producing within the last 300 years more and more secondary symptoms and indeed so many that at least seven-eighth of all the chronic maladies spring from it as their only source while the remaining eighth springs from **syphilis** and **sycosis**."[478]

All diseases except sexually transmitted diseases are due to **psora**, Hahnemann said. He did not mention how **psora** causes these diseases. Neither did he mention pathogenesis nor the different specific **aetiological** agent. Hahnemann also did not describe features of **psora** and he also did not give any evidence except a hypothesis. He gave a list of diseases and said all these are due to hypothetical **psora**. He said, "So great a flood of numberless nervous trouble, painful ailments, spasms, ulcers (cancers), adventitious formations, dyscrasias, paralysis, consumptions and crippling of soul, mind and body were never seen in ancient times when the **psora** mostly confined itself to its dreadful cutaneous symptoms of leprosy. Only during the last few centuries has mankind been flooded with these infirmities owing to the causes just mentioned. It was thus the **psora** became the most universal mother of chronic diseases."[479]

List of symptoms given by Hahnemann caused by **psora** are: "Vertigo, dizziness, rush of blood to head, heat in the head, headache, roaring noise in the brain, dandruff, eruption on the head, **tinea capitis**, baldness, paleness, redness of face, **erysipelas**, **inflammation of eye**, **dropsy** of eye, **cataract**, **squint**, **far-sightedness**, **short-sightedness**. **double vision**, **night blindness**, **amaurosis**, running pulsation and various sounds in the ear, deafness, swelling of the parotid gland, **epistaxis**, **polypi** of the nose, sense of smell perverted, redness and swelling of lips, gum disease, toothache, looseness of teeth, coated tongue, inflammation and bitter taste in mouth, **eructations,** heart burn, water brash, nausea, vomiting, cough, hiccough, ravenous hunger, appetite without hunger, spasm in stomach, distension of abdomen, tired and sleepy, headache, after meals, pain inabdomen, colic, hardness of abdomen, uterine spasm, **inguinal hernias**, **constipation**, **diarrhoea**, problems about stool, **haemorrhoids, polypi in the rectum**, pain, full retention of urine, erosion in the anus and the **perinaeum,** urine of different colours, diabetes, sexual problems, disappearance of testicles, **impotency**, **sterility**, enlargement ofprostate gland, menstrual disorder, **polypi** in the vagina, leucorrhoea, **coryza**, **laryngo bronchial phthisis**, **aphony** and hoarseness of voice, cough, **whooping cough**, pain in chest, nightmare, **asthma**, suffocation, palpitation, excessive enlargement of breast, pain in the back, burning and itching in the heal and soles, painful swollen joints, softening of bones, curvature of the spine, fragility of bone, intolerable pain and numbness of the skin, varices, **whitlow**, **paronychia, chilblains, corns, boils, furuncle**, ulcers, tumefaction and suppuration of the **humerus**, the femur, patella, bone of fingers and toes; eruptions, **warts**, encysted tumors in the skin and cellular tissue, perspirations, faintness, **tetanus**, **tremor**, loss of consciousness, **epilepsy**, **insomnia**, **somnambulism**, intermittent fever, disturbance of the mind and spirit of all kinds, anxiety, mania, quick change of mood, disinclination to work."[480]

"These are the symptoms, observed by me (Hahnemann) which, if they are often repeated or become constant, show the internal **psora** is coming forth from its latent state"[481], said Hahnemann.

At the time of Hahnemann there was no knowledge regarding **aetiological** agents, pathogenesis, clinical **symptomatology**, clinical diagnosis, investigations and natural prognosis that's why Hahnemann presumed by mistake that all diseases are due to **psora** without giving specific names to diseases.

Every person suffers from some kind of health problem in his life. And this is also true that every person also suffers with some skin manifestations in his lifetime. Hahnemann correlated these two events and said every disease except sexually transmitted disease is due to **psora** which is represented in body by external skineruptions during the latent state. Hahnemann also said by mistake that when skin eruptions subside severe manifestations result. He also said that **psora** spreads from one person to another.

The above description was written by Hahnemann in the following words:

"The itch disease is however also the most contagious of all chronic **miasmata,** far more infectious than the other two chronic miasmata the **venereal chancre** disease and the **figwart disease**. To effect the infection with the latter there is required a certain amount of friction in the most tender parts of the body which are the most richest in nerves and covered with the thinnest cuticle, as in the genital organs unless the miasma should touch a wounded spot. But the miasma of the itch needs only to touch the general skin especially with tender children. The disposition of being affected with the miasma of the itch is found with almost everyone and under almost all circumstances, which is not thecase with the other two miasmata."[482]

When **psora** spreads from one person to another person then what happens? Hahnemann writes ,"As soon as the miasma of itch *e.g.* touches the hand, in the moment when it has taken effect it no more remains local. Henceforth all washing and cleansing of the spot avail nothing. Nothing is seen on the skin during the first days, it remains unchanged and according to appearance, healthy. Living organism then has been penetrated by this specific excitation until the change of the whole being to a man thoroughly **psoric** and thus the internal development of the **psora** has reached completion."[483]

When internal development of **psora** has been completed then what will be the position of health? Body is diseased or body remains healthy.

Hahnemann says, "Only when the whole organism feels itself transformed by this peculiar chronic miasmatic disease, the diseased vital force endeavors to alleviate and to soothe the internal malady through the establishment of a suitable local symptom on the skin, the itch vesicles. So long as this eruption continues in its normal form the internal **psora**, with its secondary ailments cannot break forth but must remain covered, slumbering, latent and bound."[484]

These eruptional symptoms work as a substitute for the internal malady and keeps the **psora** in confined and stable position.

Hahnemann also said **herpes** and **tinea capitis** were external representation ofinternal **psora**. "These alone can propagate this disease to other persons because they alone contain the communicable **miasm** of **psora**."[485] Hahnemann did not know this fact that **herpes** is a viral infection and **tinea capitis** is a fungal infection. He thought that bothare different manifestations of**psora**.

50

Slumbering and bound *psora* break out due to improper treatment by Allopathic physician, through some unlucky physical or psychical occurrence, through a violent fright, through continual vexations, deeply affecting grief, through catching a severe cold or through a cold temperature, etc. Suppression of itch is mainly responsible for awakening of internal **psora** which gives many chronic **symptomatology** and diseases.

ARGUMENT

Now there is a question, how does this slumbering and bound **psora** awake and outbreak? Hahnemann answers this question. Hahnemann says, "Most of all through weakening and exhausting improper treatment by Allopathic physicians."[486] The other causes of awakening of **psora** as mentioned by Hahnemann are—

"The eruption of itch by no means remains as persistently in its place on the skin as the **chancre** and **figwart**. Even if the eruption of itch has not (as is nearly always the case) been driven away from the skin through the faulty practice of physicians and quacks by means of desiccating washes, *sulphur ointments*, drastic purgatives or cupping. It frequently disappears as we say of itself *i.e.* through causes which are not noticed. It often disappears through some unlucky physical or physical occurrence through a violent fright, through continual vexations, deeply affecting grief, through catching a severe cold or through a cold temperature, through cold, lukewarm and warm river baths or mineral bath, by a fever arising from any cause or through a different acute disease, through persistent **diarrhoea**, sometimes also perhaps through a peculiar want of activity in the skin and the results in such a case are just as mischievous as if the eruption had been driven away externally by the irrational practice of a physician. The secondary ailments of the internal **psora** and anyone of the innumerable chronic diseases flowing from this origin will then breakout sooner or later."[487] Eruption of itch is suppressed by Allopathic physicians and other causes as mentioned by Hahnemann in reference no. 487. suppression of itch is mainly responsible for awakening of internal **psora** which gives many chronic **symptomatology** and diseases.

The main concept of Homeopathy regarding **psora** and chronic diseases is suppression of itch. Hahnemann said—

"**Psora** manifests itself when the external local symptoms which serves to assuage the internal malady is hastily removed.... The diseases partly acute but chiefly chronic springing from such a one sided destruction of the chief skin symptoms (eruptions and itching) which acts vicariously and assuage the internal **psora**."[488]

Hahnemann said again and again that all chronic diseases are due to suppression of eruption and itch. How suppression of itch transformed into diseases, he said nothing. What are the characteristic features of **psora**, he also said nothing.

Hahnemann quoted observation of Ludwig Christian Juncker in support of suppression of itch and origin of diseases. "He observed that with young people of a sanguine temperament, the suppression of itch is followed by **phthisis** and with persons in general who are of a sanguine temperament, it is followed by **piles**, haemorrhoidal colic and renal gravels; with persons of sanguine choleric temperament by swelling of the inguinal glands, stiffening of the joints and malignant ulcers; with fat persons by a suffocating catarrh and mucous consumption also by inflammatory fever, **acute pleurisy** and inflammation of lungs. **Plegmatic** persons in consequence of such suppressions suffered chiefly from **dropsy**, menses were delayed and when the itch was driven away during their flow they were changed into a monthly **hemoptysis**. Persons inclined to **melancholy** were sometimes made insane by such repression, if they were pregnant the foetus was usually killed. Sometimes the suppression of itch causes sterility."[489] Now it is clear that in Homeopathy bad thinking leads to origin of **psora** which "for many thousands of years had disfigured and tortured mankind and which during the last centuries has become the mother of all the thousands of incredibly various (acute) and chronic (non-venereal) diseases."[490] This is the main concept of Homeopathy which is absolutely wrong.

51

Hahnemann presented a list of 97 examples of different clinical manifestations and proved by simple observation of appearance and disappearance of lesions that all clinical problems were due to suppression of itch. There are 15 examples in the list where suppression of **tinea** complex results in secondary diseases.

ARGUMENT

Now I will explain how Hahnemann reached the wrong conclusion of suppression of itch and origin of diseases.

At that time there was no knowledge regarding aetiology and pathogenesis of diseases. According to his own knowledge and imagination hypothesis was established without experimental studies. Hahnemann said, "The causes of all diseases are **psora**, **syphilis** and **sycosis**. **Psora** is mother of all diseases." It was an imagination of Hahnemann. Most of the cases of **syphilis** and **sycosis** were cured spontaneously. Hahnemann thought that he was curing the diseases by only a single dose of drug with dilutions up to 10^{60}. As I have already written, many diseases are cured spontaneously that's why different pathies get false reputation as an effective therapy. Homeopathy also got such a false reputation and became popular. Hahnemann developed the concept of **psora** for non-venereal diseases. Spontaneous cure of **syphilis** and **sycosis** gave false confidence to Hahnemann regarding his work. Concept of **psora** was based on wrong conclusions which derived by observing one or two cases of different diseases. Hahnemann never did controlled study in many patients. He made a very simple statement that "presence of **psora** in the body is represented by itch or skin eruptions and suppression of itch is responsible for secondary manifestations of many chronic diseases."

Medical facts cannot be deduced on the basis of only one or two examples. This mistake was committed by Hahnemann and his followers. Hahnemann writes, "Eruption of itch also disappears through catching a severe cold or through a cold temperature." [491] In support of this conclusion he instructed to see observation no. 67. In this observation, "A man whose **tinea capitis** had passed off from intense cold was seized after eight days with a malignant fever with vomiting accompanied at last with hiccough. He died in consequence on the ninth day."[492]

Hahnemann presented a list of 97 examples of different clinical manifestations and proved by simple observation of appearance and disappearance of lesions that all clinical problems were due to suppression of itch.

In example no. 5, it is mentioned that "a boy of 13 years having suffered from his childhood with **tinea capitis**, had his mother remove it for him but he became very sick within 8 or 10 days, suffering from **asthma**, violent pain in the limbs, back and knee whichwere not relieved until an eruption of itch broke out over his whole body a monthlater."[493]

There are 25 examples in the list where suppression of **tinea capitis infection** results in secondary clinical manifestations.

In example 5, suppression of **tinea capitis** results in **asthma**. In example 6, **tinea capitis** was driven away by purgative and produced symptoms of cough and lassitude. In example 16, suppression of **tinea capitis** produced fever and in other examples produced blood in skull, petrified brain, swelling of the glands of neck, violent fever, pain in back, headache were also due to suppression of **tinea capitis**.

Hahnemann says that **tinea capitis** is not a localized disease. He also says, "Localized disease is not possible. According to him, all localized lesions are external manifestations of generalized disease. Without general involvement local lesions are not possible." But Hahnemann was wrong, it can be explained very well.

Tinea infection is a fungus infection and it is localized without general involvement. **Scabies**, **boils**, **carbuncle**, **contact dermatitis**, **pityriasis versicolor,** localized candid infection, skin carcinomas are also localized lesions.

Tinea capitis is a chronic fungal infection. Acquisition of a fungal infection (**dermatophyte**) appears to be favoured by minor trauma, maceration and poor hygiene of the skin. Usually **dermatophytes** infections are cured spontaneously due to reason given here. "Invasion of the stratum corneum by **dermatophytes** (ringworm or **tinea**) may cause little inflammation or particularly with zoophilicfungi inflammation can be intense. Shedding of the stratum corneum is increased by inflammation, to the extent that fungal growth cannot keep up with shedding. Inflammation may help terminate infection. Conversely infection is probably favoured when shedding is reduced by **corticisteroids** and cytotoxic drugs."[494] Today, through knowledge of medical science we know that suppression of **tinea capitis** can never produce any other disease. **Asthma**, fever, pain can never be produced by suppression of **tinea.** It was a wrong observation by Hahnemann. Suppression of **tinea** was neither related with development of **asthma,** fever or other manifestations nor reappearance of **tinea** infection was related with cure of these diseases. It was just coexistence of two different diseases and nothing else.

In the list of observations "Hahnemann quoted 13 examples of **asthma**"[495] and he concluded that suppression of**tinea**/rash/itch resulted in **asthma** and reappearance ofskin lesions again resulted in recovery. If skin lesions are not appeared again then there is possibility of death as mentioned in example 15 and example 70. Facts about **asthma** were not known to Hahnemann. He though that asthma was due to suppression of itch, rash or **tinea** and reappearance of rash or itch or**tinea** resulted in cure. But facts are as follows, "**Asthma** is manifested physiologically by a widespread narrowing of the air passage which may be relived spontaneously or as a result of therapy. Asthma is manifested clinically by paroxysms of **dyspnoea** cough and wheezing. It is an episodic disease, acute exacerbations being interspersed with symptom free period. Typically most attacks are short-lived lasting from minutes to hours and after them the patient seems to recover completely clinically"[496] and "**Allergic asthma** is frequently seasonal and it is most often observed in children and young adults. **Allergic asthma** is often associated with a personal and/or family history of **rhinitis**, **urticaria** and **eczema**. History of periodic attacks are quite characteristic. The natural course of **asthma** in adult life has been littleinvestigated. Some studies suggest that spontaneous remissions occur inapproximately 20 per cent of those who develop the disease as adults and 40 per cent or so can be expected to improve with less frequent and severe attacks as they grow older."[497]

Now it is clear that **asthma** of allergic type is usually associated with **eczema** or **urticaria** which are skin lesions. In other words skin lesions are usually associated with **allergic asthma**. Suppression of skin lesions never produce **asthma**. Another interesting fact about asthma is, "It is paroxysmal. A person who is subjected to **asthma** may be perfectly well, but one minute and half an hour later may be in the throes of a violent attack. An attack may last minutes, hours or days and when prolonged is termed as **status asthmaticus**. As the attack subsides breathing becomes gradually easier, the patient often coughs up plug of mucous sputum and then rapidly recovers. There are many interesting features in this disease such as a personal history of skin eruptions (**urticaria**, **prurigo** and **eczema**), these often alternating with paroxysms of **asthma**." [498] Regarding prognosis "Children frequently grow out of the disease about puberty. Adults never lose the tendency to attacks but may be free for years." [499]

Now we summarise the total characteristic features of **asthma**. They are—

1. Paroxysmal episodic character.
2. Free intervals of varying period between attacks.
3. Associated with skin lesions.
4. Skin eruptions are present often alternating with paroxysms of asthma.
5. Chances of spontaneous recovery.
6. Children frequently grow out of the disease about puberty.

On the basis of the above conclusions, it can be said that the conclusion derived by Hahnemann about the origin and cure of **asthma** was wrong. Origin and recovery from **asthma** is not due to appearance or suppression of eruptions.

52

Time interval is different in different cases after the suppression of itch and development of secondary disease. **Epilepsy** and fever also developed due to suppression of itch. Reappearance of itch and eruption is a must for a cure.

ARGUMENT

Hahnemann did not give any explanation about how suppression of rash creates disease. He also did not explain how only one mechanism that is suppression of itch developed different diseases in different persons. He did not say how much time it would take in development of secondary manifestations after suppression of itch. In example 75 he quoted, "A count, 57 years old, had suffered for three years with dry itch. It was driven off and he enjoyed an apparently good health for two years, only he had two attacks of vertigo during this time.... A similar attack followed six weeks later then once a month for three months."[500] In example 81, it is written, "A youth of 18 years drove off the itch with a *mercurial* ointment and two months after he was unexpectedly seized with convulsions."[501] In example 85, it is mentioned, "A youth of 18 who had driven out itch with*mercurial remedies* was seized a few weeks later with **epilepsy**, which returned after four weeks with the new moon."[502] In example 88, it is mentioned, "Five year old itch passed away and this after several years produced **epilepsy**."[503]

In example 75, 85 and 88, time interval is different in different cases after suppression of itch and development of secondary manifestations. In example 75 it is two years, in example 81 it is two months, in example 85 it is few weeks and in example 88 it is several years. In these examples in one case **epilepsy** is produced two months after suppression of itch, in other cases **epilepsy** is produced after few weeks and after several years of suppression of itch. In many cases secondary manifestations are developed soon after suppression of itch. This shows that this correlation is not accurate. In the list of 97 examples, 11 are of **epilepsy**. It has been also said about epilepsy that this originated due to suppression of itch. It is not the truth. Hahnemann should have thought how in one case **epilepsy** developed soon after suppression of itch and in other case **epilepsy** developed after many years of suppression of itch. But he did not analyse accurately. Skin eruptions, itch, skin lesions, **boil**, **acne**, **eczema**, **fungal infection** and many other skin disease are very common. Everybody suffers with one or other localized skin disease sometimes in his life. He also suffers with many other diseases. Hahnemann falsely correlated both these. "Epilepsy is a group of disorders characterized by chronic recurrent paroxysmal changes in neurological function caused by abnormal electrical activity of the brain. Causes of seizures are intracranial birth injury, acute infection, metabolic disturbances, genetic disorders, febrile convulsion, alcoholism, brain tumor, cardiovascular"[504] disease, etc. "Epileptic attacks usually recur at intervals throughout life but in some cases they disappear spontaneously either for years or permanently. Occasionally isolated fits may not be repeated."[505] "Convulsions in infancy are not necessarily followed by **epilepsy** in adult life. **Pyknolepsy** (attacks of minor epilepsy in children) is said to disappear completely at puberty. In some cases one or two fits occur in adolescence and then a long remission follows. In exceptional cases isolated major fits may occur in adult life and notrecur. Most confirmed epileptics are able to live a normal working life under selected conditions away from potential danger (machinery, furnaces, heights) and to many have healthy children."[506] We have seen that causes of **epilepsy** are not related with skin lesions and attacks of **epilepsy** are recurrent. Time interval is not fixed for recurrent attacks. Attack may recur on the same day or second attack may come after a gap of months or years. There is also the possibility that **epilepsy** may not recur at all. Then this statement that **epilepsy** occurs due to suppression of itch is absolutely wrong.

At present there is no evidence that localized treatment of skin disease causes development of secondary diseases. If Hahnemann is right then all skin specialists should be banned. There should not be provision of skin specialists according to Homeopathy, because they mainly suppress or treat localized skin lesions externally. Homeopathy says, "Skin specialists are dangerous. They create many severe secondary diseases by removing localized skin lesions."

Do you agree with this pseudo fact? Should skin specialists be banned?

There were 16 cases of fever and associated symptoms in this list. It had been said by Hahnemann that fever was due to suppression of itch and reappearance of itch or eruption is must for cure of fever, as written in example 72, "After driving off itch, most frequently acute fevers with a great sinking of the strength follows. In one such case the fever lasted for seven days, when the eruption of itch reappeared and stopped the fever."[507]

There are many diseases of fever where skin eruptions appear. But suppression of eruptions is not the cause of disease and reappearance of eruptions is not the cause of cure. Many fevers have eruptions as a sign of the disease. Eruptions are manifestations of diseases and appearance and disappearance are related stages of diseases. "Examples of such diseases are: (1) Viral infection: **rubeola, rubella**, **hepatitis**, **measles**, arboviruses, adenoviruses,**vaccinia, herpes simplex, dengue**, **yellow fever**, (2) Bacterial infection: **scarlet fever, erysipelas, sub-acute bacterial endocarditis, typhoid fever, bullous, impetigo,** gonococcemia Hemophilus influenza**, (3) Rickettsial: rocky mountain spotted fever, epidemic typhus** (4) Fungal: **candidiasis, sporotrichosis**, (5) **Chlamydial psittacosis**, (6) Protozoal: **toxoplasmosis**, **trichinosis**, (7) **Immunological**, and (8) Drug eruptions."[508]

"The pathogenesis of an exanthema may be caused by (1) Multiplication of the pathogen in the skin, (2) Carriage of the agent in plasma or in infected hematopoietic cells (leucocytes and or lymphocytes) into integumentary blood vessels, and (3) Antigen antibody or delayed hypersensitivity reactions to antigen derived from the infecting micro-organisms regional multiplication of the virus, primary viremia and visceral dissemination of virus occur prior to the development of the **exanthema** and explain why the initial clinical manifestations of many viral illnesses occur prior to the development of the rash... . In some petechial eruptions direct evidence of viral or bacterial invasion can be obtained by direct aspiration and culture of the lesion, by demonstrating of the agent with Gram's stain or by immunofluorescent stain to detect microbial agents."[509]

"Some **exanthematous** diseases produce characteristic **cutaneous** patterns... . A streptococci produces a rash that starts on the neck and spreads to the trunk and extremities within 36 hours... . The course of the eruption is also helpful in differentiating the etiology of viral **exanthemas**... . The eruption of rubella tends to disappear from its original site of involvement as it spreads... . The cutaneous lesions tend to wax and wane with fever."[510]

"In each of the acute exanthemata, the eruption has special and distinctive character which together with the day of the disease on which the eruption appears may enable one to differentiate the members of this group from one another. In **chickenpox** rash appears on the first day of pyrexia, in **scarlet fever** it appears on second day, in **smallpox** it appears on third day, in measles rash appears on the fourth day of pyrexia."[511]

Rash appears and disappears according to disease present. "In **chickenpox** within 24 hours the characteristic eruptions appear... . after a day or so skin lesions dries into a scab... . within 10 to 14 days separates, leaving a pigmented scab."[512]

"In **scarlet fever**—the rash continues to be well marked until the fourth or fifth day of the disease but disappear earlier if *antitoxin* or *penicillin* have been given... . the rash indicates the production of an **erythrogenic** toxin by the infecting organism."[513]

"In **erysipelas** the rash may vary in duration from three to four days to a fortnight and it is materially shortened by chemotherapy."[514]

"**Dengue** or **break bone fever** is a specific fever lasting for not more than seven days and mainly confined to tropical climates... . often within one to two days the skin over the face, neck and chest becomes flushed and reddened (primary rash) by the third or fourth day, the temperature falls to 100°F or lower... . the patient temporarily feels better but after a few hours to three days' temperature again rises, the pain returns and secondary rash appears and... . for lasts a few hours to three days. Desquamation and itching follows."[515]

"In **influenza** eruptions of erythematous or urticarial type occur."[516]

"In *typhoid* the rash generally appears about the seventh to twelfth day (average 10th) in successive crops of small rose coloured **lenticular** spots slightly elevated, soft and disappearing on pressure. Each spot lasts for about three to four days and they are never petechial. They are chiefly seen on the abdomen."[517]

By the above description it should be clear that skin eruptions are characteristic feature of diseases. Eruptions develop during pathogenesis of disease. Eruptions are parts of disease. Disease first enters the body then eruption develops. Suppression of eruptions do not develop disease. Appearance of eruption is not related with cure of disease.

There are various other types of fevers where rash is not present. Examples are **mumps**, **diphtheria**, **rheumatic fever**, **yellow fever**, **cat scratch fever**, **malaria amoebiasis**, etc. These fevers are not related to rash. Then there is no question of establishment of relation between suppression of itch and origin of disease.

53

Hahnemann himself quoted examples where without applying external Allopathic treatment, eruptions were suppressed and created secondary clinical symptoms.

ARGUMENT

Hahnemann said repeatedly that suppression of external lesions or eruptions by external Allopathic treatment is very dangerous and responsible for various secondary manifestations. Surprisingly he himself quoted examples where without applying external ointment eruptions were suppressed and created secondary symptoms, as written in case 64, "with a boy the itch passed away by itself, this was followed by fever."[518]

In case no. 65, "Itch disappeared from the skin of itself, on which lingering fever, expectoration of pus and lastly death followed."[519]

In example no. 78, it is written, "A girl of 17 in consequence of **tinea capitis** which disappeared by itself was seized with continuous heat in the head and attacks of headache."[520] External eruptions also went away because of the cold as mentioned in case no. 67.

"A man whose **tinea capitis** had passed off from intense cold was seized after eight days with a malignant fever with vomiting."[521]

Hahnemann emphasized mainly on removal of eruptions, figwart and **chancre** by Allopathic doctors externally and said this is a very dangerous procedure, because these suppressed eruptions and external skin lesions cause widespread secondary manifestations. Same phenomenon also occurs itself as mentioned by Hahnemann in quoted examples. When we compare both these events we find that in one group secondary manifestations were present after applying external ointment and in second group without applying external ointment secondary manifestations were also present.

By this comparison we can say that development of secondary manifestations are not related to application of external ointment. Again we can say the hypothesis of Hahnemann was wrong, conclusion of Hahnemann was wrong, Homeopathy was wrong and Homeopathy is wrong.

"These 97 examples were basis of concept of **psora**. Hahnemann repeatedly quoted these examples for various conclusions."[522] In one example (no. 91) "a woman after having the itch driven out had paralysis of one leg, in example 92 after driving offthe itch with sulphur ointment, a man of 53 years had **hemiplegia**, in example 47 driven offthe itch with ointment leads to complicated kidney problem, in example 27, it caused death and whole of lung was filled with liquid pus, in example 30 diaphragm and the liver were diseased, in example 34 it caused death, in example 44 bleeding piles, in example 17 bloody **expectroration**, **dyspnoea**, and death etc."[523]

As written in above references, according to Hahnemann suppression of itch by itself or by application of external ointment are mainly responsible for secondary manifestations. Hahnemann did not give any mechanism how suppression leads to secondary diseases. He also did not explain which patient would suffer with what type of ailments after suppression of eruptions. He also did not do controlled experiments.

54

New medicine and new dose of the same medicine would interrupt the work of improvement and cause new ailments which often cannot be repaired for a long time. If somebody does this, he is unworthy of a Homeopathic physician. In exceptional cases, repetition of dose is allowed but in different potency. Homeopathic drugs are effective also by respiratory route. When the treatment of infant is concerned, Hahnemann advised drug administration to nursing mother.

ARGUMENT

Hahnemann writes regarding frequency of doses—"the disease of it be not one of very long standing will generally be removed and extinguished by the first dose of it without any considerable disturbance."[524]

He also writes, "Every perceptibly progressive and strikingly increasing amelioration during treatment is a condition which, as long as it lasts, completely precludes every repetition of the administration of any medicine in more chronic diseases, a single dose of an appropriate selected Homeopathic remedy will in time complete but slowly, with progressive improvement and give the help which such a remedy in such a case can accomplish naturally within 40, 50, 60, 100days."[525] "It is impractical to repeat the same unchanged dose of a remedy once, not to mention its frequent repetition. The vital principle does not accept such unchanged dose without resistance." [526] "The physician must therefore in chronic diseases allow all antipsoricremedies to act 30, 40 or even 50 and more days by themselves, so long as they continue to improve the diseased state perceptibly to the acute observer, eventhough gradually, for so long the good effects continue with the indicated doses these must not be disturbed and checked by any new remedy."[527] Why did Hahnemann oppose repetition of same dose of medicine? He said, "a second dynamically wholly similar unchanged dose of the same medicine no longer finds, therefore the same condition ofthe vital force. The patient may indeed be made sick in another way by receiving other such unchanged doses, even sicker than he was, for now only those symptoms of the given remedy remain active which were not Homeopathic to the original disease, hence no step towards cure can follow, only a true aggravation of the condition of the patient."[528]

Hahnemann made a fundamental rule in the treatment of chronic diseases. "To let the action of the remedy selected in a mode Homeopathic, appropriate to the case of disease which has been carefully investigated to its symptoms, come to an undisturbed conclusion, so long as it visibly advances the cure and the while improvement still perceptibly progress. This method forbids any new prescription, any interruption by another medicine and forbids as well immediate repetition of the same remedy."[529] He said, new medicine and new dose of the same medicine would interrupt the work of improvement and cause new ailments which often cannot be repaired for a long time. He writes, "Still there has been of late much abuse of this immediate repetition of doses of the same medicine, because young Homeopaths thought it more convenient to repeat, without examination, a medicine which in the beginning had been found to beHomeopathically suitable."[530] "We may declare at once, that the practice of late which has even been recommended in public journals, of giving the patient several doses of the same medicine to take with him, so that he may take them himself at certain intervals, without considering whether this repetition may affect him injuriously seems to show a negligent empiricism and to be unworthy of a Homeopathic physician, who should not allow a new dose of a medicine to be taken or given without convincing himself in every case before hand as to its usefulness."[531] Hahnemann advised, "Repetition of the same medicine in exceptional cases where beneficial remedy has made some beginning toward an improvement but its action ceases too quickly, its power is too soon exhausted and the cure does not proceed any further. This is rare in chronic diseases but in acute diseases and in chronic diseases that rise into an acute state, it is frequently the case but this repetition should be permitted only when the preceding dose has largely exhausted its action (after six, eight or ten days) and the dose should be just as small as the preceding one and be given in a different potency."[532]

Homeopathy says, a single dose of Homeopathic drug is effective orally and sufficient for complete cure in chronic diseases. These drugs are also effective when taken through respiratory route. "If only a small vial say a dram of dilute *alcohol* is used in the treatment, in which is contained and dissolved through succussion one globule of the medicine which is to be used by olfaction every two, three or four days, this also must be thoroughly succussed eight to ten times before each olfaction."[533] "By such an inhalation the power of any **potentized** medicine may be communicated to the patient in any degree of strength such medicated pellets kept in a stoppered vial retain their medicinal power quite undiminished, even if the vial be preserved from sunshine and heat."[534] "Even persons born without the sense of smell or who have lost it through disease, may expect equally efficient help from drawing in the imperceptible vapour through one nostril or the other, as those do who are gifted with the sense of smell. From this it follows the nerves possessing merely the sense 'touch' receive the salutary impression and communicate unfailingly to the whole nervous system."[535] When treatment of child is concerned, Hahnemann advised drug administration to the nursing mother. He said, "the power of medicines acting upon the infant through the milk of the mother of wet nurse is wonderfully helpful. Every disease in a child yields to the rightly chosen homoeopathic medicines given in moderate doses to the nursing mother and so administered, is more easily and certainly utilized by these new world citizens then is possible in later years. Since most usually have imparted to them **psora** through the milk of the nurse, if they do not already possess it through heredity from the mother they may be at the same time protected antipsorically by means of the milk of the nurse rendered medicinally in this manner."[536] Here Hahnemann said, "Single dose of Homeopathic drug is sufficient in chronic diseases." There is no necessity of repetition of the drug. Effect lasts up to 50 or more days. In acute diseases drug can be repeated only in different potency. Same drug with similar potency should not be repeated in

Homeopathy. If such a drug is repeated then the drug will be harmful. For this conclusion there is no experimental study in Homeopathy. At present Homeopaths themselves do not follow this rule of Hahnemann. They use drugs in frequent doses with similar potency as they desire without any logics. Followers of Homeopathy themselves are against the rules of Hahnemann. See the statement of Hahnemann which is highly ridiculous, illogical and irrelevant. He says at one place for the treatment of infants that drug should be given to nursing mother as mentioned in reference no. 536. Actually what happened in spontaneously curable self-limiting diseases, whatever methods applied by Hahnemann, he thought that he had been able to treat the diseases successfully. In this way he made a wrong concept of Homeopathy.

55

Hahnemann accepted failure of Homeopathic treatment. He said that he was not able to cure all chronic patients. He mentioned many factors which made patients incurable and augmented their diseases.

ARGUMENT

Hahnemann got curative results in **syphilis** and **sycosis** by Homeopathic method of treatment because these diseases are cured spontaneously. He was convinced wrongly that he had been curing these patients. For remaining diseases he made other group of **psora** and he observed many case history of patients showing prejudice and applied Homeopathic law of treatment without doing controlled experiment.

Fatal disease are those diseases where death is certain, if not properly treated. There is no possibility of spontaneous recovery in fatal diseases. All patients of fatal diseases will definitely die if treatment is not available. Acquired Immuno-Deficiency Syndrome (AIDS) is a fatal illness caused by a retrovirus. **Rabies**, also known as **hydrophobia** is an acute highly fatal viral disease. These are two communicable diseases of man that are always fatal. Tropical diseases like **malaria**, **fevers**, **typhoid**, **cholera**, **dysentery**, **amoebiasis**, **measles**, **chickenpox** are not fatal diseases. In the absence of proper treatment patients may die or recover spontaneously.

Maximum number of patients with tropical diseases, if not treated recover spontaneously due to immunity in the body. Only few patients die if not effectively treated. Without effective treatment recovery may take a longer time *e.g.* **typhoid** is cured spontaneously within a month in the absence of treatment but presence of effective treatment cures **typhoid** within a week. "Without effective antibiotic treatment **typhoid fever** kills almost 10 per cent of those infected."[537]

Case fatality rate represents the killing power of a disease. It is simply the ratio of deaths to cases. The time interval is not specified. The case fatality rate for the same disease may vary in different epidemics because of changes in the agent, host and environmental factors. "Case fatality is closely related to virulence.

$$\text{Case fatality ratio (rate)} = \frac{\text{Total number of deaths due to a particular disease}}{\text{Total number of cases due to same disease.}"^{538}} \times \frac{100}{1}$$

"**Measles** is a viral infection. In a developing country case fatality rate ranges from 2 to 15 per cent."[539] This indicates 2 to 15 deaths per 100 patients without treatment in **measles**. "In **typhoid**, case mortality varies in different epidemics from 5 to 20 per cent."[540] "**Hepatitis B** is a systemic viral infection. Usually it is an acute self-limiting infection. In approximately 5 to 15 per cent of cases it fails to resolve and the affected individual then becomes a persistent carrier of the virus."[541] "In one study case fatality rate of **hepatitis B** was 15.6 per cent."[542]

In **lobar pneumonia**, if patients are not treated by antibiotic and then "the fever persists at 104° or 105°F for an average of seven to eight days. The patient continues to be extremely ill with a hot dry skin, a painful cough, considerable sleeplessness and exhaustion and takes little nourishment. About the seventh or eighth day the fever as also the pulse and respiration rate, in favourable cases terminate by crisis falling to normal in the course of a few hours. This is accompanied by marked general improvement, the pulse respiration ratio returns to normal.

Conclusively we can say in tropical diseases maximum number of patients recover spontaneously without effective treatment but may take longer duration. A small per cent of patients may die in tropical diseases without treatment. We can get 100 per cent cure rate if diseases are treated properly. In non-tropical diseases like **hypertension**, **diabetes**, **cancer**, **asthma**, etc. if diseases are not treated properly then there is gradual deterioration and death but this may take years. In non-tropical diseases like **myocardial infarction, cardiac failure**, **cerebral stroke**, **kidney failure**, patients die sooner or later in the absence of treatment.

In chronic diseases there is possibility of fluctuation in severity. Remissions and exacerbations are also there. Without clinically controlled trials these fluctuations give wrong impression of cure.

A percentage of population react positively to placebo. "A placebo is a vehicle for cure by suggestion and surprisingly often successful if it is only temporary. All treatment carry placebo effect. A placebo reactor is an individual who reports change of physical or mental state after taking a pharmacologically inert substance. Such suggestible people are likely to respond favourably to any treatment. They have deceived doctors into making false therapeutic reputations. Some 35 per cent of the physically ill and 40% of mentally ill respond to placebo."[544]

Non-tropical diseases like cardiac problems, **diabetes**, **renal diseases**, **carcinomas**, **strokes** usually begin in elderly people. Children, adolescent and young persons usually do not suffer from these diseases. They suffer mainly from tropical diseases which usually resolve spontaneously in large number of patients.

Hahnemann put all non-sexually transmitted diseases in one group and said they are due to **psora**. He prescribed different **antipsoric** Homeopathic drugs for different diseases according to the Homeopathic principle. He said, "The eruption is only to be removed by internal healing and curative remedies which change the state of the whole, then also the eruption which is based on the internal disease will be cured and healed of itself without the help of any external remedy and frequently more quickly than it could be done by external remedies."[545] He also said, "The great truth is established that all chronic ailments, all great and the greatest, long continuing disease (excepting the few venereal ones) spring from **psora** alone and only find their thorough cure in the cure of **psora**; they are consequently to be healed mostly only by **antipsoric** remedies *i.e.* by those remedies which in their provings as to their pure action on the healthy human body manifest most of the symptoms which are most frequently perceived in latent as well as in developed **psora**."[546]

Hahnemann thought all diseases are due to **psora**, **syphilis** and **sycosis.** He wrongly accepted that he was able to cure diseases by Homeopathic method. The fact was not obvious to Hahnemann. He did not have knowledge about pathology, aetiology, diagnosis and treatment of disease. He also did not know— "Clinical evaluation of a drug and how drug is discovered."

More than 70 per cent patients suffer from tropical diseases and 70 to 80 per cent of patients suffering from tropical disease are cured spontaneously without any effective treatment. It is certain that without effective treatment some patients may die and in remaining patients morbidity, severity and duration of disease will be greater. By the help of modern medical effective treatment morbidity, severity and duration of disease are decreased with cent per cent cure. Spontaneous recovery in large per cent of population gave wrong message to the world that Homeopathy is effective. Similar unnecessary reputation is also being earned on similar grounds by many useless therapies like Ayurveda, magnet, religion, tantra-mantra, etc.

Placebo reaction also gives transitory curative effect which helps in the establishment of reputation of unnecessary and useless pathies. To understand the fact that Homeopathy is fraud, knowledge of medical science is must. If a person is glorifying any pathy after seeing curative effect in one or two patients, it means he does not know anything regarding medical science. If a medical specialist like M.B.B.S. praises Homeopathy or any other empirical therapy, it means he is ignorant. He should be debarred from practicing medicine being guilty of spreading and advancing spurious learning.

That's why I say Hahnemann was wrong. Homeopathy was wrong. Homeopathy is wrong. It works as placebo only. Homeopathy has no therapeutic utility

Hahnemann accepted failure. He said that he was not able to cure all chronic patients. He also said, "Homeopathy is ineffective if there are certain conditions." What are those factors, which make Homeopathy ineffective. These are:

"Hahnemann said these events if they occur in a person who is already a chronic patient may not only augment his disease and increase the difficulty of curing it but if they break in on him violently may make his disease incurable, if the untoward circumstances are not suddenly changed for the better."[547]

- He writes about failure in effectiveness of Homeopathic treatment "An innocent man with less injury to his life can pass 10 years in bodily torments in the **bastile** or on the galleys rather than pass some months in all bodily comfort..." [548] Why? What are those factors which increase duration of disease and decrease effectiveness of Homeopathic treatment? He writes—"Excessive hardships labouring in swamps, great bodily injury and wounds, excess of cold and heat and even the unsatisfied hunger of poverty and its unwholesome foods"[549] are the causes which prolong duration of disease in an innocent man.

- According to Hahnemann, contempt and poverty are also responsible for producing chronic ailments. He says, "A **psora** slumbering within which still allows the favourite of a prince to live with the appearance of almost blooming health unfolds quickly into a chronic ailment of the body or distracts his mental organs into insanity."
- How does **suppuration of the lung** or **cancer of the breast** develop? Hahnemann answers, "The sudden death of a son causes the tender mother, already in ill health, an incurable **suppuration of the lungs** or a **cancer of the breast**."[551]
- Hahnemann accepted unsuccess in the treatment in following words, "How difficult it is and how seldom will the best anti-**psoric** treatment do anything to relieve such unfortunates?"[552] He says all imaginable chronic sufferings can develop from uninterrupted grief and vexation. "If grief and vexation continually beatin upon him and it is out of the power of the physician to effect a lasting removal of these most active destroyers of life, he had better give up the treatment and leave the patient to his fate for even the most masterly management of the case with the remedies that are the most exquisite and the best adopted to the bodily ailment will avail nothing, nothing at all, with a chronic patient thus exposed to continue sorrow and vexation."[553] Hahnemann agreed that grief and vexation prevent curative effect of Homeopathic drugs. Even it has been said by Hahnemann that "It is better to leave the patient to his fate rather than to treat when patient is in grief and vexation." Vexation means a state of being annoyed and worried. When a person is in severe chronic ailments he would be definitely in grief and vexation. Hahnemann says this patient cannot be cured. According to him first grief and vexation should be removed then disease will be cured. But this is not the fact. The fact is that first disease should be removed then grief and vexation will subside automatically.
- Hahnemann rationalized failure of treatment. He produced unnecessary pretence... . When diseases have been cured spontaneously, he gave credit to Homeopathy. When diseases have not been cured he made responsible those factors which were not actually responsible for failure. For example in reference no. 551he said **suppuration of lung** and **cancer of breast** are incurable due to sudden death of son of patient. Today a person having knowledge of diseases knows very well that death of a son cannot be made responsible for incurable **suppuration of lung** and **carcinoma of breast**. In this way we can say Hahnemann accepted failure but

produced wrong arguments. Conclusively, we can say that grief and vexation cannot make disease incurable, if successful treatment is available. Hahnemann says such things which indicates only failure of Homeopathic treatment.

- Other causes of incurability of chronic diseases, as mentioned by Hahnemann are— "Almost as near and often nearer yet to incurability are the chronic diseases especially with great and rich men who for some years besides the use of mineral bath, passed through the hands of various often of many allopathic physicians. And after the continuation of such irrational medical assaults on the organism for several years, it becomes almost quite incurable."[554] I agree that old Allopathic treatment was injurious to health and blood of thepatient was made to flow by bleeding, leeches, etc. or medicine was prescribed to evacuate the contents of stomach and intestine. These procedures destroyed the life acutely but after the gap of a considerable time things were changed. Toxic and harmful effect of old Allopathic treatment should have disappeared aftersometime. If Homeopathic treatment was effective then it could have cured these patients. They should have been managed by Homeopathic treatment. But Hahnemann was not able to manage these patients and he illogically projected mineral bath and allopathic treatment as causes of failure.
- Other causes of failure of Homeopathic treatment are ridiculous. Hahnemann writes—"Great hindrance to a cure of far advanced chronic diseases is often found in the debility and weakness into which youth fall who are spoiled by richparents, being carried away by their superabundance and wantonness and seduced by wicked companions through destructive passions and excesses through revealing abuse of the sexual instinct, gambling, etc. without the least regard for life and for conscience bodies originally robust are debilitate by such vices into mere semblances of humanity."[555]

  This paragraph says that if the patient is a gambler or spoiled youth of rich parents, cannot be treated by Homeopathic treatment.
- Hahnemann also mentioned a typical cause of failure. This cause is not related to patient but this cause is related to disease. He says that "there is nevertheless found at times, especially with the lower classes of patients a peculiar obstruction to the cure, which lies in the source of the malady itself where the **psora** after repeated infections and a repeated external repression of the resulting eruptions had developed gradually from its internal state into one of "[556] more severe chronic ailments. He also writes, "if patients are aged or debilitated, chances of improvement are very less."[557]

- Here Hahnemann writes very clearly that if disease is chronic then chances of improvement are very rare. If patients are aged or debilitated then chances of cure are less. It shows Hahnemann himself admits that chances of failure ofHomeopathic treatment are very high.
- Prescription of new drug or repetition of same medicine also interfere recovery. As Hahnemann says—"Once a medicine because it was selected in a correct Homeopathic manner is acting well of usefully, which is seen by the 8th or 10th day... The dose will then probably have exhausted its favourable action about the 40th or 50th day and before that time it would be injudicious and an obstruction to the progress of the cure to give any other medicine"[558] and "the whole treatment will amount to nothing. Another antipsoric remedy which may be ever so useful, but is prescribed too early and before the cessation of the action of the present remedy or a new dose of the same remedy which is still usefully acting can in no case replace the good effect which has been lost through the interruption of the complete action of the preceding remedy which was acting usefully which can hardly be again replaced."[559] In some cases "every new medicine and also a new dose of the same medicine would interrupt the work of improvement and cause new ailments, an interference which often cannot be repaired for a long time."[560] If a Homeopath gives new **antipsoric** medicine or repeats same medicine within 30 or 40 days of first dose in treatment of chronic diseases, it will be the definite cause of failure of treatment, says Hahnemann. He says repetition of dose of same medicine or new drug in chronic diseases will interfere in recovery or creates new diseases, if used within 30 or 40 days. Followers of Homeopathy use frequent doses. They are against Hahnemann. Are they treating patients or they are creating new ailments? Can you answer?
- Hahnemann also provided a list of conditions which disturb the treatment. He enumerated "overloading the stomach, disorder of the stomach from fat, nausea and inclination to vomit, disorder of the stomach with gastric fever, chilliness and cold, fright and timidity, vexation, sadness caused by the fright, vexation which causesanger, heat irritation, indignation with silent internal mortification, unsuccessful love with quite grief, unhappy love with jealousy, a severe cold, a cold which is followed by suffocative fits, cold followed by pains and inclination to weep, cold with consequent **coryza**, contusions and wounds inflicted by blunt instruments, burning of the skin, weakness from loss of fluids and blood, homesickness with redness of the cheeks."[561]

These are the conditions which also interfere treatment.

- Hahnemann also says that large or strong dose of a drug also creates hurdles in treatment. He says, "A medicine even though it may be Homeopathically suited to the case of disease, does harm in every dose that is too large and in strong doses it does more harm, the greater its Homeopathically and higher the potency selected and it does much more injury than any equally large dose of a medicine that is unhomeopathic and in no respect adapted to morbid state (allopathic). Too large doses of an accurately chosen Homeopathic medicine and especially whenfrequently repeated bring about much trouble as a rule."[562]
- Hahnemann also advised many precautions which should be taken during Homeopathic treatment otherwise treatment will not be effective. He said, "obstacles to cure is so much the more necessary in the case of patients affected by chronic diseases, as their diseases are usually aggravated by such noxious influences and other diseases, causing errors in the diet and regimen which often pass unnoticed."[563] These are "coffee, Chinese and other herb teas,beer... all kind of punch, spiced chocolate, odorous waters and perfumes of many kinds, strong scented flowers in the apartment, tooth powders, and essences and perfumed sachets, compounds of drug, highly spiced dishes and sauces, spiced cakes and ices,... all vegetables possessing medicinal properties, celery, onions, old cheese... heated rooms, woollen clothing next the skin, a sedentary life in close apartments or the frequent indulgence in mere passive exercise (such as riding, driving or swinging), prolonged suckling, taking a long siesta in a recumbent posture in bed, sitting up long at night, uncleanliness, unnatural debauchery, enervation by readingobscene books, reading while lying down, onanism or imperfect or suppressed intercourse in order to prevent conception, subjects of anger, grief or vexation, a passion for play, over-exertion of mind or body especially after meals, dwelling in marshy districts, damp-rooms, penurious living etc. All these things must be as far as possible avoided or removed, in order that the cure may not be obstructed or rendered impossible."[564]
- Hahnemann also mentioned astronomical influence. He writes, "During the treatment of chronic diseases by antipsoric remedies we often need the other non-antipsoric store of medicines in cases where epidemic diseases or intermediate arising usually from meteoric and telluric causes attack our chronic patient and so not only temporarily disturb the treatment but even interrupt it for a longer time."[565]

- Hahnemann mentioned many factors for failure of Homeopathic treatment. It is not correct. Reality is different from what has been said by Hahnemann.

Actually, I am now explaining what the fact was.

The diseases which resolved spontaneously Hahnemann gave the credit to Homeopathy. Diseases which were not resolved spontaneously were attributed to many other factors. Whatever he observed in patients gambling, onions, perfumes, flowers, tooth powders, vegetables, meteoric body, rest and sleep taken in the early afternoon, grief and vexation etc, interfere in Homeopathic treatment. A person with knowledge of science and diseases knows very well that these factors mentioned by Hahnemann do not influence recovery of diseases. In fact Hahnemann was wrong. Homeopathy has only placebo effect.

Homeopathy got good results only in those patients who were being deteriorated by old Allopathic methods especially in acute **pyrexial** and in **acute diarrhoeal diseases**. In these cases actually Homeopathy was not effective but old Allopathic methods had to be stopped which were dangerous and fatal to patients suffering from acute feverish and **acute diarrhoeal diseases**. In management of **smallpox**, "fluid deficit should be replaced by administration of appropriate solutions." [566] In treatment of **typhoid,** "nursing care and attention to nutritional requirements are important. Laxative and enemas should be avoided."[567]

In dysentery, "A fluid or semi-fluid, low roughage diet should be given depending on the severity of **diarrhoea** but if this is severe, it will be necessary to replace the *water* and *electrolyte* loss by intravenous therapy."[568]

In **whooping cough** "when the illness is of long duration and vomiting is frequent, skilled nursing will be required to maintain nutrition, especially in infants and young children."[569]

When a person is suffering from fever and **diarrhoea** adequate nutrition and water electrolyte balance are very necessary to prevent morbidity and mortality. If dehydration is produced in these patients by vomiting and purgation and blood is removed from the body then these procedures become highly dangerous and detrimental to the body and increase morbidity and mortality. Then chances ofspontaneous recovery are over. In **measles, cholera, scarlet fever, whooping cough, dysentery** and **typhoid**, chances of spontaneous recovery are great. When in these patients dehydration is produced or blood is removed, chances of complications and death are very much increased. In these patients Homeopathic method did not provide cure but protected the patients from damaging effect of old Allopathy, prevalent at that time. That's why Homeopathy got a reputation as a curing agent. Hahnemann writes—"**small-pox measles**, purple rash, **scarlet fever, whooping cough**, **dysentery** and **typhoid** when they complete their course especially without a judicious Homeopathic treatment, leave the organism so shaken and irritated.... This is due to the great exhaustion of the organism which still commencement of the correct treatment even to the restoration of health and of the normal state. The strength increases during the use of so called tonics and the patients joyously rises up again of themselves in proportion as their life as delivered from its corroding enemy."[571] But the fact is "Homeopathy itself has no therapeutic ability, but replaced old Allopathy that's why Homeopathy prevented exhausting debilitating effect of old Allopathy and got false reputation as a curative and highly effective therapeutic method."

Nowadays the concept of old Allopathy has totally changed. Today, developed medical science is based on scientific study, experiments and controlled observations. Purgation, blood removal and concept of plethora are not accepted today. Electrolytes and fluid are administered in dehydrated conditions and blood is also administered when required. Knowledge of different branches of science is being used today in the medical field. New advanced methods of investigation are being used today. Morbidity and mortality are also reducing day by day. Today we have a vast knowledge. Acceptance of Homeopathy indicates our ignorance, lack of knowledge, unscientific approach and inability to understand science and knowledge. Prevalence of Homeopathy in 2007 A.D. is against the society, against humanity, and against the intelligence. Societies and nations are losing money, time and lives by supporting Homeopathy.

The aim of this work was to analyse mistakes done by Hahnemann. Now we know that Hahnemann made many mistakes. Now there is also no doubt that Homeopathy has no therapeutic effect. Whatever beneficial effect obtained by Homeopathic drugs is actually a placebo effect. We have also discussed that placebo therapeutic effect is psychological and such an effect can be obtained by inert substances.

Many standard text books of modern medical science and clinical trials also support my conclusion that Homeopathic drugs have no therapeutic effect.

H.P. Rang, M.M. Dale, J.M. Ritter, P.K. Moore write in Pharmacology—"Hahnemann introduced the practice of Homeopaathy in the early 19th century. The system rapidly drifted in to absurdity... . Public acceptance, alas has little to do with demonstrable efficacy."[572]

D.R. Laurence, P.N. Bennett, M.J. Brown mention in *Clinical Pharmacology*—Pharmacologists generally feel that in the absence of conclusive evidence from empirical studies that Homeopathic medicines can reproducibly be shown to differ from placebo in clinical studies conducted according to modern scientific standards, there is no point in discussing the hypotheses of Homeopathy.[573]

In *Applied Pharmacology* by Walter Modell, Heinz Schield, Andrew Wilson, it is mentioned that "Hahnemann's system of Homeopathy rapidly drifted in to absurdities. Homeopathy was devoid of any scientific basis."[574]

R.S. Satoskar and S.D. Bhandarkar write in *Pharmacology & Pharamacotherapeutics* regarding Homeopathy—"The claims are, however difficult to understand in the light of present concept of diseases, nor can they be substantiated by various scientific methods applied to the study of modern medicine."[575]

"In a highly reputed medical journal **Lancet**, recently an analysis of clinical trials of Homeopathic drugs has been published",[576] which clearly declares Homeopathic drugs are no better than a placebo. Swiss scientists compared the result of more than 100 trials of Homepathic medicines with the same number of trials of conventional medicines in a range of conditions. They found that Homeopathy had no more than placebo effect. An editorial written in the **Lancet** titled "The End of Homeopathy" demands that doctors recognize the absence of real curative powers in Homepathic medicine. This editorial also says "it is more surprising that the debate continue after 150 years of unfavourable findings."[576]

The aim of this work was to analyse mistakes done by Hahnemann. Now we have known that Hahnemann made many mistakes. Now there is also no doubt that Homeopathy has no thereapeutic effect. Whatever beneficial effect obtained by Homeopathic drugs is actually a placebo effect. We have also discussed that placebo therapeutic effect is a psychological effect and such effect can be obtained by inert substances.

At one time Homeopathy protected the public from ill effects of old Allopathic treatment. At present Homeopathy is misguiding the public and increasing morbidity and mortality because it is interfering in application of modern medical science.

That's why:
Homeopathy should be discarded.
Homeopathy should be banned.
Homeopathy has no curative ability.
Homeopathy has no therapeutic utility.
It is an illusion only.

NOTES

1. James Coleman. *Abnormal Psychology and Modern Life*. Taraporewala and Sons, Bombay, 1976, 27.
2. Remington. *The Science and Practice of Pharmacy,* Vol. II, 20th edition, Alfanso Gennaro, William and Wilkins, Baltimore, 2000, 1771.
3. D.R. Laurence, P.N. Bennet. *Clinical Pharmacology*, E.L.B.S., 6th edition, Churchill, Livingstone, UK, 1983, 27.
4. Satoskar, Bhandarka. *Pharmacology and Pharmacotherapeutics,* 11th edition, Bombay Popular Prakashan, 1988, 1.
5. Modell, Schield Wilson. *Applied Pharmacology.* American edition, W.B. Saunders Company, Toronto, 1976, 9.
6. Krantz and Carr. *The Pharmacological Principles of Medical Practice,* 6th edition, Williams and Wilkins Company, Baltimore, 1965, 158.
7. Dipalma, Joseph. *Drill's Pharmacology in Medicine,* 3rd edition, McGraw Hill Book Company, New York, 1965, 1388.
8. F. Dualey Hart. *French's Index of Differential Diagnosis*, 12th edition, Wrigh-London, 1985, 737.
9. Herbert French. *An Index of Differential Diagnosis of Main Symptoms*, 6th edition, Bristol, Johnwright, London, 1945, 744.
10. Petersdorf, Adams, Braunwald. *Harrison's Principle of Internal Medicine* 10th edition. McGraw Hill, 1983, New Delhi, 1190-1195.
11. F. Dudley Hart. *French's Index of Differential Diagnosis,* 12th edition, Wright, London, 1985, 285.
12. Satoskar, Bhandarkar. *Pharmacology and Pharmacotherapeutics.* Bombay Popular Prakashan, 11th edition, 1988, 655.
13. K. Park. *Park's Textbook of Preventive and Social Medicine,* 15th edition, Banarsidas Bhanot Publishers Jabalpur, 1997, 188 and 193.
14. *Op. cit.,* 5.

15. *Ibid.*

16. Alfred Goodman Gilman, Louis Goodman, Alfred Gilman. *Goodman & Gilman's Pharmacological Basis of Therapeutics*, 6th edition, Macmillan, Newyork, 1980, 1623.

17. N.J. Modi. *Textbook of Medical Jurisprudence and Toxicology*, 9th edition, N.M. Tripathi Publishers Bombay, 1975, 545.

18. N.J. Modi. *Textbook of Medical Jurisprudence and Toxicology*. 9th edition, N.M. Tripathi Publishers, Bombay, 1975, 551.

19. Krantz and Carr. *The Pharmacological Principles of Medical Practice,* 6th edition, Williams and Wilkins Company, Baltimore, 1965, 206.

20. Alfred Goodman Gilman, Louis Goodman, Alfred Gilman. *Goodman & Gilman's Pharmacological Basis of Therapeutics*, 6th edition, Macmillan, New York, 1980, 1624.

21. Charles, Craig and Robert Stitzel. *Modern Pharmacology,* 2nd edition, 1986, Little Brown, USA, 515.

22. Charles, Craig and Robert Stitzel. *Modern Pharmacology*, 2nd edition, 1986, Little Brown, USA, 544.

23. *Op. cit.,* 5.

24. *Op. cit.,* 5.

25. Doordarshan DD-1, U.G.C. Programme, 6-7 A.M. Date 26.6.2002.

26. Samuel Hahnemann. *Organon of Medicine* (English) Translated by William Boericke. B. Jain Publishers (P) Ltd., New Delhi - 110 055, 6th edition, 1993, 15-17.

27. Samuel Hahnemann. *Organon of Medicine* (English) Translated by William Boericke. B. Jain Publishers (P) Ltd., New Delhi - 110 055, 6th edition, 1993, 17.

28. Samuel Hahnemann. *Organon of Medicine* (English) Translated by William Boericke. B. Jain Publishers (P) Ltd., New Delhi - 110 055, 6th edition, 1993, 162, Paragraph 74.

29. Samuel Hahnemann. *Organon of Medicine* (English) Translated by William Boericke. B. Jain Publishers (P) Ltd., New Delhi - 110 055, 6th edition, 1993, pp. 75 -76, 163-64.

30. Samuel Hahnemann. *Organon of Medicine* (English) Translated by William Boericke. B. Jain Publishers (P) Ltd., New Delhi – 110 055, 6th edition, 1993, Paragraphs, 1, 92.

31. Samuel Hahnemann. *Organon of Medicine* (Hindi) Translated by Prabha Devi. B. Jain Publishers (P) Ltd., New Delhi 1996, 30.

32. Samuel Hahnemann. *Organon of Medicine* (English) Translated by William Boericke. B. Jain Publishers (P) Ltd., New Delhi – 110 055, 6th edition, 1993, 97.

33. Samuel Hahnemann. *Organon of Medicine* (Hindi) Translated by Prabha Devi. B. Jain Publishers (P) Ltd., New Delhi, 1996, Paragraphs 13, 37.

34. James Kent. *Lectures on Homeopathic Philosophy*. B. Jain Publishers (P) Ltd., New Delhi - 110 055, 1993, 22.

35. James Kent. *Lectures on Homeopathic Philosophy*. B. Jain Publishers (P) Ltd., New Delhi - 110 055, 1993, 34.

36. Petersdorf, Adams, Braunwald. *Harrison's Principle of Internal Medicine,* 10th edition. McGraw Hill, New Delhi, 1983.

37. Alfred Goodman Gilman, Louis Goodman, Alfred Gilman. *Goodman & Gilman's Pharmacological Basis of Therapeutics*, 6th edition, Macmillan, New York, 1980, 1085-94.

38. Alfred Goodman Gilman, Louis Goodman, Alfred Gilman. *Goodman & Gilman's Pharmacological Basis of Therapeutics*, 6th edition, Mackmillan, New York, 1980, 1081.

39. Alfred Goodman Gilman, Louis Goodman, Alfred Gilman. *Goodman & Gilman's Pharmacological Basis of Therapeutics*, 6th edition, Macmillan, New York, 1980, 1085.

40. Alfred Goodman Gilman, Louis Goodman, Alfred Gilman. *Goodman & Gilman's Pharmacological Basis of Therapeutics*, 6th edition, Macmillan, New York, 1980, 1100.

41. J.R. Anderson. *Muir's Textbook of Pathology,* E.L.B.S., 12th edition, 1985, Edward Arnold London - Introduction.

42. *Ibid.*

43. J.R. Anderson. *Muir's Textbook of Pathology,* E.L.B.S., 12th edition, 1985, Edward Arnold London - Introduction.

44. *Ibid.*

45. K. Park. *Park's Textbook of Preventive and Social Medicine,* 15th edition, Banarsidas Bhanot Publishers, Jabalpur, 1997, 85.

46. Samuel Hahnemann. *Organon of Medicine* (English) Translated by William Boericke. B. Jain Publishers (P) Ltd., New Delhi - 110 055, 6th edition, 1993, Paragraphs 18, 21.

47. Samuel Hahnemann. *Organon of Medicine* (Hindi) Translated by Prabha Devi. B. Jain Publishers (P) Ltd., New Delhi 1996, 41.

48. Petersdorf, Adams, Braunwald. *Harrison's Principle of Internal Medicine*, 10th edition, McGraw Hill, 1983, New Delhi, 58.

49. Samuel Hahnemann. *Organon of Medicine* (English) Translated by William Boericke. B. Jain Publishers (P) Ltd., New Delhi - 110 055, 6th edition, 1993, Paragraphs 18, 70, 156-57.

50. Samuel Hahnemann. *Organon of Medicine* (English) Translated by William Boericke. B. Jain Publishers (P) Ltd., New Delhi - 110 055, 6th edition, 1993, p. 18, Paragraphs 19, 106.

51. Samuel Hahnemann. *Organon of Medicine* (English) Translated by William Boericke. B. Jain Publishers (P) Ltd., New Delhi - 110 055, 6th edition, 1993, Paragraphs 18, 22, 107.

52. Samuel Hahnemann. *Organon of Medicine* (Hindi) Translated by Prabha Devi. B. Jain Publishers (P) Ltd., New Delhi 1996, Paragraph 18.

53. Samuel Hahnemann. *Organon of Medicine* (English) Translated by William Boericke, B. Jain Publishers (P) Ltd., New Delhi - 110 055, 6th edition, 1993, Paragraphs 18, 21, 107.

54. Samuel Hahnemann. *Organon of Medicine* (English) Translated by William Boericke. B. Jain Publishers (P) Ltd., New Delhi - 110 055, 6th edition, 1993, Paragraphs 18, 27, 112.
55. Samuel Hahnemann. *Organon of Medicine* (English) Translated by William Boericke. B. Jain Publishers (P) Ltd., New Delhi - 110 055, 6th edition, 1993, Paragraphs 18, 24, 109.
56. Alfred Goodman Gilman, Louis Goodman, Alfred Gilman. *Goodman & Gilman's Pharmacological Basis of Therapeutics*, 6th edition. Macmillan, New York, 1980, 1085.
57. Satoskar, Bhandarkar. *Pharmacology and Pharmacotherapeutics,* Bombay Popular Prakashan, 11th edition, 1988, 1.
58. Samuel Hahnemann. *Organon of Medicine* (Hindi) Translated by Prabha Devi. B. Jain Publishers (P) Ltd., New Delhi, 1996, Paragraphs 34, 116.
59. Samuel Hahnemann. *Organon of Medicine* (English) Translated by William Boericke. B. Jain Publishers (P) Ltd., New Delhi - 110 055, 6th edition, 1993, pp. 18, 38, 118.
60. W.A.D. Anderson *Pathology*, Vol. 1, 6th edition, C.V. Mosby© Company, St. Louis, 1971, 376.
61. J.R. Anderson. *Muir's textbook of Pathology*, 10th edition, E.L.B.S., 1976, 161.
62. J.R. Anderson. *Muir's textbook of Pathology*, 10th edition, E.L.B.S., 1976, 162.
63. Petersdorf, Adams, Braunwald. *Harrison's Principle of Internal Medicine*, 10th edition, McGraw Hill, 1983, New Delhi, 1095.
64. J.R. Anderson. *Muir's Textbook of Pathology*, 10th edition, E.L.B.S., 1976, 162.
65. Samuel Hahnemann. *Organon of Medicine* (Hindi) Translated by Prabha Devi. B. Jain Publishers (P) Ltd., New Delhi 1996, 124.
66. Samuel Hahnemann. *Organon of Medicine* (English) Translated by William Boericke. B. Jain Publishers (P) Ltd., New Delhi - 110 055, 6th edition, 1993, pp. 38, 120.
67. *Ibid.*
68. Samuel Hahnemann. *Organon of Medicine* (English) Translated by William Boericke. B. Jain Publishers (P) Ltd., New Delhi - 110 055, 6th edition, 1993, pp. 46, 129.
69. *Ibid.*
70. *Ibid.*
71. Samuel Hahnemann. *Organon of Medicine* (English) Translated by William Boericke. B. Jain Publishers (P) Ltd., New Delhi - 110 055, 6th edition 1993, pp. 46, 129.
72. Samuel Hahnemann. *Organon of Medicine* (English) Translated by William Boericke. B. Jain Publishers (P) Ltd., New Delhi - 110 055, 6th edition, 1993, pp. 79-80, 166-67.

73. Samuel Hahnemann. *Organon of Medicine* (English) Translated by William Boericke. B. Jain Publishers (P) Ltd., New Delhi - 110 055, 6th edition, 1993, pp. 104, 187.

74. Samuel Hahnemann. *Organon of Medicine,* (English) Translated by William Boericke. B. Jain Publishers (P) Ltd., New Delhi - 110 055, 6th edition, 1993, p. 190.

75. Samuel Hahnemann. *Organon of Medicine* (English) Translated by William Boericke. B. Jain Publishers (P) Ltd., New Delhi - 110 055, 6th edition, 1993, pp. 105-06, 109, 187-89.

76. Samuel Hahnemann. *Organon of Medicine* (English) Translated by William Boericke. B. Jain Publishers (P) Ltd., New Delhi - 110 055, 6th edition, 1993, pp. 110, 191.

77. Samuel Hahnemann. *Organon of Medicine* (English) Translated by William Boericke. B. Jain Publishers (P) Ltd., New Delhi - 110 055, 6th edition, 1993, pp. 18, 128, 201.

78. Samuel Hahnemann. *Organon of Medicine* (English) Translated by William Boericke. B. Jain Publishers (P) Ltd., New Delhi - 110 055, 6th edition, 1993, Paragraph 18, pp. 129, 202.

79. Samuel Hahnemann. *Organon of Medicine* (English) Translated by William Boericke. B. Jain Publishers (P) Ltd., New Delhi - 110 055, 6th edition, 1993, Paragraphs 18, 115, 194.

80. Samuel Hahnemann. *Organon of Medicine* (English) Translated by William Boericke. B. Jain Publishers (P) Ltd., New Delhi - 110 055, 6th edition, 1993, Paragraph 18, pp. 131, 203.

81. Samuel Hahnemann. *Organon of Medicine* (English) Translated by William Boericke. B. Jain Publishers (P) Ltd., New Delhi - 110 055, 6th edition, 1993, pp. 18, 134, 205.

82. Samuel Hahnemann. *Organon of Medicine* (Hindi) Translated by Prabha Devi. B. Jain Publishers (P) Ltd., New Delhi 1996, pp. 136, 139.

83. D.R. Laurence and P.N. Bennett. *Clinical Pharmacology.* E.L.B.S. with Churchill Livingstone, 7th edition, 1992, 120-21.

84. *Ibid.*

85. James Tyler Kent. *Lecture on Homeopathic Philosophy.* B. Jain Publishers (P) Ltd., Delhi, 1993, 186.

86. Samuel Hahnemann. *Organon of Medicine* (English) Translated by William Boericke. B. Jain Publishers (P) Ltd., New Delhi - 110 055, 6th edition, 1993, Paras 63, 149.

87. Samuel Hahnemann. *Organon of Medicine* (English) Translated by William Boericke. B. Jain Publishers (P) Ltd., New Delhi - 110 055, 6th edition, 1993, Paras 64, 150.

88. Samuel Hahnemann. *Organon of Medicine* (English) Translated by William Boericke. B. Jain Publishers (P) Ltd., New Delhi - 110 055, 6th edition, 1993, Paras 11, 98.

89. Samuel Hahnemann. *Organon of Medicine* (English) Translated by William Boericke. B. Jain Publishers (P) Ltd., New Delhi - 110 055, 6th edition, 1993, Paras 31, 50.

90. Samuel Hahnemann. *Organon of Medicine* (English) Translated by William Boericke. B. Jain Publishers (P) Ltd., New Delhi - 110 055, 6th edition, 1993, 52.

91. William Ganong. *Review of Medical Physiology* 10th edition. Prentice-Hall International, Appleton & Lange, U.S.A., 1999, 44-45.

92. Guyton and Hall. *A Textbook of Medical Physiology,* 10th edition. W.B. Saunders Company, Philadelphia, 2000, 7-8.

93. Samuel Hahnemann. *Organon of Medicine* (English) Translated by William Boericke. B. Jain Publishers (P) Ltd., New Delhi - 110 055, 6th edition, 1993, Paras 26, 111.

94. Samuel Hahnemann. *Organon of Medicine* (English) Translated by William Boericke. B. Jain Publishers (P) Ltd., New Delhi - 110 055, 6th edition, 1993, Paras 27, 112.

95. Satoskar, Bhandarkar. *Pharmacology and Pharmacotheapeutics.* Bombay Popular Prakashan, Mumbai, 11th edition, 1988, 102.

96. Samuel Hahnemann. *Organon of Medicine* (English) Translated by William Boericke. B. Jain Publishers (P) Ltd., New Delhi - 110 055, 6th edition, 1993, Para 28, 112.

97. Samuel Hahnemann. *Organon of Medicine* (English) Translated by William Boericke. B. Jain Publishers (P) Ltd., New Delhi - 110 055, 6th edition, 1993, Paras 45, 128.

98. Samuel Hahnemann. *Organon of Medicine* (Hindi) Translated by Prabha Devi. B. Jain Publishers (P) Ltd., New Delhi 1996, Paras 34, 52.

99. Samuel Hahnemann. *Organon of Medicine* (English) Translated by William Boericke. B. Jain Publishers (P) Ltd., New Delhi - 110 055, 6th edition, 1993, Paras 48, 133.

100. Samuel Hahnemann. *Organon of Medicine* (English) Translated by William Boericke. B. Jain Publishers (P) Ltd., New Delhi - 110 055, 6th edition, 1993, Paras 68, 153.

101. Samuel Hahnemann. *Organon of Medicine* (Hindi) Translated by Prabha Devi. B. Jain Publishers (P) Ltd., New Delhi 1996, Paras 68, 89-90.

102. Samuel Hahnemann. *Organon of Medicine* (English) Translated by William Boericke. B. Jain Publishers (P) Ltd., New Delhi - 110 055, 6th edition, 1993, Paras 155, 219.

103. Samuel Hahnemann. *Organon of Medicine* (English) Translated by William Boericke. B. Jain Publishers (P) Ltd., New Delhi - 110 055, 6th edition, 1993, Paras 68, 153.

104. Samuel Hahnemann. *Organon of Medicine* (Hindi) Translated by Prabha Devi. B. Jain Publishers (P) Ltd., New Delhi 1996, Paras 69, 91.

105. Samuel Hahnemann. *Organon of Medicine* (Hindi) Translated by Prabha Devi. B. Jain Publishers (P) Ltd., New Delhi 1996, Paras 29, 49.

106. Samuel Hahnemann. *Organon of Medicine* (Hindi) Translated by Prabha Devi. B. Jain Publishers (P) Ltd.,, New Delhi 1996, pp. 107, 112, 122. Samuel Hahnemann. *Organon of Medicine* (English) Translated by William Boericke. B. Jain Publishers (P) Ltd., New Delhi - 110 055, 6th edition, 1993, Paras 93, 112.

107. Samuel Hahnemann. *Organon of Medicine* (Hindi) Translated by Prabha Devi. B. Jain Publishers (P) Ltd., New Delhi 1996, pp. 63, 85.

108. Rosa Waugh Hobhouse. *Life of Christian Samuel Hahnemann.* World Homeopathic Links, New Delhi - 110 055, 1984, 78.

109. Rosa Waugh Hobhouse. *Life of Christian Samuel Hahnemann.* World Homeopathic Links, New Delhi - 110 055, 1984.

110. Krantz and Carr. *The Pharmacological Principles of Medical Practice*, 6th edition. Williams and Wilkins Company, Baltimore 1965, 205-06.

111. Wilson, Schild and Modell. *Applied Pharmacology.* E.L.B.S. Churchill Livingstone, London 11th edition, 1975, 550.

112. Wilson, Schild and Modell. *Applied Pharmacology*. E.L.B.S. Churchill Livingstone, London 11th edition, 1975, 234.

113. Wilson, Schild and Modell. *Applied Pharmacology*. E.L.B.S. Churchill Livingstone, London 11th edition, 1975, 410.

114. Alfred Goodman Gilman, Louis Goodman, Alfred Gilman. *Goodman & Gilman's Pharmacological Basis of Therapeutics*, 6th edition, Macmillan, 1980, 1623-25.

115. Petersdorf, Adams, Braunwalk. *Harrison's Principle of Internal Medicine*, 10th edition, McGraw Hill, 1983, New Delhi, 1034-40.

116. W.A.D. Anderson. *Pathology*, Vol. 1, 6th edition. C.V. Mosby Company, St. Louis, 1971, 209-12.

117. W.A.D. Anderson. *Pathology,* Vol. 1, 6th edition. C.V. Mosby Company, St. Louis, 1971, 350-52.

118. Rosa Waugh Hobhouse. *Life of Christian Samuel Hahnemann*. World Homeopathic Links, New Delhi - 110 055, 1984, 131.

119. *Ibid.*

120. Samuel Hahnemann. *Organon of Medicine* (English) Translated by William Boericke. B. Jain Publishers (P) Ltd., New Delhi - 110 055, 6th edition, 1993, Paras 158, 221.

121. Samuel Hahnemann. *Organon of Medicine* (English) Translated by William Boericke. B. Jain Publishers (P) Ltd., New Delhi - 110 055, 6th edition, 1993, Paras 157, 220.

122. Satoskar, Bhandarkar. *Pharmacology and Pharmacotherapeutics.* Bombay Popular Prakashan, 11th edition, 1988, 121.

123. Samuel Hahnemann. *Organon of Medicine* (English) Translated by William Boericke. B. Jain Publishers (P) Ltd., New Delhi - 110 055, 6th edition, 1993, 221-22.

124. Alfred Goodman Gilman, Louis Goodman, Alfred Gilman. *Goodman & Gilman's Pharmacological Basis of Therapeutics,* 6th edition, Macmillan, New York, 1980, 980-81.

125. Rosa Waugh Hobhouse. *Life of Christian Samuel Hahnemann.* World Homeopathic Links, New Delhi - 110 055, 1984, 135-36.

126. James Coleman. *Abnormal Psychology & Modern Life*. Taraporewala & Sons, Bombay.

127. Talbott, Hales, Yudofsky. *Textbook of Psychiatry*. American Psychiatric Press, 1988, 414.

128. Krantz and Carr. *The Pharmacological Principles of Medical Practice*, 6th edition, Williams and Wilkins Company, Baltimore 1965, 692.

129. Rosa Waugh Hobhouse. *Life of Christian Samuel Hahnemann*. World Homeopathic Links, New Delhi - 110 055, 1984, 142-43.

130. Rosa Waugh Hobhouse. *Life of Christian Samuel Hahnemann*. World Homeopathic links, New Delhi - 110 055, 1984, 143.

131. *Ibid.*

132. Rosa Waugh Hobhouse. *Life of Christian Samuel Hahnemann*. World Homeopathic Links, New Delhi - 110 055, 1984, 145.

133. Alfred Goodman Gilman, Louis Goodman, Alfred Gilman. *Goodman & Gilman's Pharmacological Basis of Therapeutics*, 6th edition, Macmillan, New York 1980, 980-81.

134. W.A.D. Anderson. *Pathology,* Vol. 1, 6th edition, C.V. Mosby Company, St. Louis, 1971, 287.

135. W.A.D. Anderson. *Pathology,* Vol. 1, 6th edition, C.V. Mosby Company, St. Louis, 1971, 273.

136. W.A.D. Anderson. *Pathology,* Vol. 1, 6th edition, C.V. Mosby Company, St. Louis, 1971, 274.

137. Ronald Bodley Scott. *Price's Textbook of Practice of Medicine*, 2nd edition, E.L.B.S. and Oxford University Press, Walton Street, Oxford 1978, 67.

138. Rains & Ritchie. *Bailey & Love's Short Practice of Surgery,* 17th edition, H.K. Lewis & Comp., 1977, 101.

139. Rosa Waugh Hobhouse. *Life of Christian Samuel Hahnemann*. World Homeopathic Links, New Delhi - 110 055, 1984, 146.

140. *Ibid.*

141. P.L. Soni. *Text book of Inorganic Chemistry*, Sultan Publications, India, 2.141.

142. P.L. Soni. *Textbook of Inorganic Chemistry*. Sultan Publications, India, 2.154.

143. P.L. Soni. *Textbook of Inorganic chemistry*. Sultan Publications, India, 3.311.

144. N.J. Modi. *Textbook of Medical Jurisprudence and Toxicology*, 9th edition, N.M. Tripathi Publisher, Bombay, 1975, 521.

145. P.L. Soni. *Textbook of Inorganic Chemistry*. Sultan Publications, India, 3.95 and 3.96.
146. Rosa Waugh Hobhouse. *Life of Christian Samuel Hahnemann*. World Homeopathic Links, New Delhi-110 055, 1984, 150.
147. *Ibid.*
148. P.L. Soni. *Textbook of Physical Chemistry*. O.P. Dharmendra, Sultan Chand & Sons, 23, Daryaganj, New Delhi, 13th revised edition, 1981, 2:82.
149. Rosa Waugh Hobhouse. *Life of Christian Samuel Hahnemann*. World Homeopathic Links, New Delhi-110 055, 1984, 241.
150. Rosa Waugh Hobhouse. *Life of Christian Samuel Hahnemann.* World Homeopathic Links, New Delhi-110 055, 1984, 82-83.
151. Rosa Waugh Hobhouse. *Life of Christian Samuel Hahnemann*. World Homeopathic Links, New Delhi-110 055, 1984, 242.
152. *Ibid.*
153. Rosa Waugh Hobhouse *Life of Christian Samuel Hahnemann*. World Homeopathic Links, New Delhi-110 055, 1984, 249.
154. K. Park. *Park's Textbook of Preventive and Social Medicine*, 15th edition, Banarsidas Bhanot Publishers, Jabalpur, 1997, 163-70.
155. Petersdorf, Adams, Braunwald. *Harrison's Principle of Internal Medicine*, 10th edition, McGraw Hill, 1983, New Delhi, 997-98.
156. Samuel Hahnemann. *Organon of Medicine*. (English) Translated by William Boericke. B. Jain Publishers (P) Ltd., New Delhi - 110 055, 6th edition, 1993, 15.
157. Dr. Neelmani Ghatak. *Cause and Cure of Chronic Diseases*. Translator Chandra Shekhar Pathak. Publisher Dr. S.M. Bhattacharya, D.M.S. Kolkata F.P.T., Alipur, Kolkata - 700053, 4th edition, 1-2.
158. Dr. Neelmani Ghatak. *Cause and Cure of Chronic Diseases*. Translator Chandra Shekhar Pathak, Publisher Dr. S.M. Bhattacharya, D.M.S. Kolkata F.P.T., Alipur, Kolkata - 700053, 4th edition, 4-7.
159. Dr. Neelmani Ghatak. *Cause and Cure of Chronic Diseases*. Translator Chandra Shekhar Pathak, Publisher Dr. S.M. Bhattacharya, D.M.S. Kolkata F.P.T., Alipur, Kolkata - 700053, 4th edition, 7.
160. Dr. Neelmani Ghatak. *Cause and Cure of Chronic Diseases*. Translator Chandra Shekhar Pathak, Publisher Dr. S.M. Bhattacharya, D.M.S. Kolkata F.P.T., Alipur, Kolkata - 700053, 4th edition, 7-9.
161. Dr. Neelmani Ghatak. *Cause and Cure of Chronic Diseases*. Translator Chandra Shekhar Pathak, Publisher Dr. S.M. Bhattacharya, D.M.S. Kolkata F.P.T., Alipur, Kolkata - 700053, 4th edition, 14-15.
162. Petersdorf, Adams, Braunwald. *Harrison's Principle of Internal Medicine*. 10th edition, McGraw Hill, 1983, New Delhi, 964-66.
163. Petersdorf, Adams, Braunwald *Harrison's Principle of Internal Medicine*. 10th edition, McGraw Hill, 1983, New Delhi, 885-89.

164. Dr. Neelmani Ghatak. *Cause and Cure of Chronic Diseases*. Translator Chandra Shekhar Pathak, Publisher Dr. S.M. Bhattacharya, D.M.S. Kolkata F.P.T., Alipur, Kolkata - 700053, 4th edition, 15.

165. Dr. Neelmani Ghatak. *Cause and cure of Chronic Diseases*. Translator Chandra Shekhar Pathak, Publisher Dr. S.M. Bhattacharya, D.M.S. Kolkata F.P.T., Alipur, Kolkata - 700053, 4th edition, 20-21.

166. *Ibid.*

167. Dr. Neelmani Ghatak. *Cause and Cure of Chronic Diseases*. Translator Chandra Shekhar Pathak, Publisher Dr. S.M. Bhattacharya, D.M.S. Kolkata F.P.T., Alipur, Kolkata - 700053, 4th edition, 21.

168. Dr. Neelmani Ghatak. *Cause and Cure of Chronic Diseases*. Translator Chandra Shekhar Pathak, Publisher Dr. S.M. Bhattacharya, D.M.S. Kolkata F.P.T., Alipur, Kolkata - 700053, 4th edition, 22.

169. Dr. Neelmani Ghatak. *Cause and Cure of Chronic Diseases*. Translator Chandra Shekhar Pathak, Publisher Dr. S.M. Bhattacharya, D.M.S. Kolkata F.P.T., Alipur, Kolkata - 700053, 4th edition, 37.

170. Dr. Neelmani Ghatak. *Cause and Cure of Chronic Diseases*. Translator Chandra Shekhar Pathak, Publisher Dr. S.M. Bhattacharya, D.M.S. Kolkata F.P.T., Alipur, Kolkata - 700053, 4th edition, 45-46.

171. K. Park. *Park's Textbook of Preventive and Social Medicine.* 15th edition, Banarsidas Bhanot Publisher Jabalpur, 1997, 117-18.

172. Samuel Hahnemann. *Organon of Medicine* (English) Translated by William Boericke. B. Jain Publishers (P) Ltd., New Delhi - 110 055, 6th edition, 1993, Paragraphs 76, 164-65.

173. Dr. Neelmani Ghatak. *Cause and Cure of Chronic Diseases*, Translator Chandra Shekhar Pathak, Publisher Dr. S.M. Bhattacharya, D.M.S. Kolkata F.P.T., Alipur, Kolkata - 700053, 4th edition, 58.

174. Samuel Hahnemann. *Organon of Medicine* (English) Translated by William Boericke. B. Jain Publishers (P) Ltd., New Delhi - 110 055, 6th edition, 1993, Paragraphs 80, 168.

175. Samuel Hahnemann. *Organon of Medicine* (English) Translated by William Boericke. B. Jain Publishers (P) Ltd., New Delhi - 110 055, 6th edition, 1993, Paragraphs 81, 169.

176. Samuel Hahnemann. *Organon of Medicine* (English) Translated by William Boericke. B. Jain Publishers (P) Ltd., New Delhi - 110 055, 6th edition, 1993, Paragraphs 78, 166.

177. Samuel Hahnemann. *Organon of Medicine* (English) Translated by William Boericke. B. Jain Publishers (P) Ltd., New Delhi - 110 055, 6th edition, 1993, 79, 80.

178. Samuel Hahnemann. *Organon of Medicine* (English) Translated by William Boericke. B. Jain Publishers (P) Ltd., New Delhi - 110 055, 6th edition, 1993, Paragraphs 194, 236.

179. *Ibid.*

180. Samuel Hahnemann. *Organon of Medicine* (English) Translated by William Boericke. B. Jain Publishers (P) Ltd., New Delhi - 110 055, 6th edition, 1993, pp. 195, 237.

181. Samuel Hahnemann. *Organon of Medicine* (English) Translated by William Boericke. B. Jain Publishers (P) Ltd., New Delhi - 110 055, 6th edition, 1993, pp. 199, 239.

182. Samuel Hahnemann. *Organon of Medicine* (English) Translated by William Boericke. B. Jain Publishers (P) Ltd., New Delhi - 110 055, 6th edition, 1993, pp. 80, 168.

183. Samuel Hahnemann. *Organon of Medicine* (English) Translated by William Boericke. B. Jain Publishers (P) Ltd., New Delhi - 110 055, 6th edition, 1993, pp. 200, 240.

184. Petersdorf, Adams, Braunwald. *Harrison's Principle of Internal Medicine,* 10th edition, McGraw Hill, 1983, New Delhi, 1174-75.

185. Samuel Hahnemann. *Organon of Medicine* (English) Translated by William Boericke. B. Jain Publishers (P) Ltd., New Delhi - 110 055, 6th edition, 1993, pp. 201, 240.

186. Samuel Hahnemann. *Organon of Medicine* (English) Translated by William Boericke. B. Jain Publishers (P) Ltd., New Delhi - 110 055, 6th edition, 1993, pp. 202, 242.

187. *Ibid.*

188. Samuel Hahnemann. *Organon of Medicine* (English) Translated by William Boericke. B. Jain Publishers (P) Ltd., New Delhi -110 055, 6th edition, 1993, Paragraphs 203, 242.

189. Samuel Hahnemann. *Organon of Medicine* (English) Translated by William Boericke. B. Jain Publishers (P) Ltd., New Delhi -110 055, 6th edition, 1993, 244.

190. Samuel Hahnemann. *Organon of Medicine* (Hindi) Translated by Prabha Devi. B. Jain Publishers New Delhi 1996, Paras 228, 198.

191. James Coleman. *Abnormal Psychology & Modern Life*. Taraporewala and Sons, Bombay, 1976, 25-36.

192. Samuel Hahnemann. *Organon of Medicine* (English) Translated by William Boericke. B. Jain Publishers (P) Ltd., New Delhi - 110 055, 6th edition, 1993, pp. 215-16.

193. Kalpan and Sadock. *Comprehensive Textbook of Psychiarty*, 4th edition, Williams & Wilkins, U.S.A., 1985, 838-50.

194. Samuel Hahnemann. *Organon of Medicine* (English) Translated by William Boericke. B. Jain Publishers (P) Ltd., New Delhi - 110 055, 6th edition, 1993, Paras 221, 253.

195. N.J. Modi. *Textbook of Medical Jurisprudence and Toxicology,* 9th edition, N.M. Tripathi Publisher Company, 1975, 742.

196. N.J. Modi. *Textbook of Medical Jurisprudence and Toxicology,* 9th edition, N.M. Tripathi Publisher Company, 1975, 697.

197. Alfred Goodman Gilman, Louis Goodman, Alfred Gilman. *Goodman & Gilman's Prarmacological Basis of Therapeutics*, 6th edition, Macmillan ,1980, 1624.

198. Kalpan and Sadock. *Comprehensive Textbook of Psychiarty*, 4th edition. Williams & Wilkins, U.S.A., 1985, 848.

199. James Coleman. *Abnormal Psychology & Modern Life*. Taraporewala and Sons, Bombay, 460.

200. Samuel Hahnemann. *Organon of Medicine* (English) Translated by William Boericke. B. Jain Publishers (P) Ltd., New Delhi - 110 055, 6th edition, 1993, Paras 270, 290-93.

201. Samuel Hahnemann. *Organon of Medicine* (English) Translated by William Boericke. B. Jain Publishers (P) Ltd., New Delhi - 110 055, 6th edition, 1993, 294.

202. Remington. *The Science and Practice of Pharmacy*, 20th edition ,Vol. II. ALFANSO–R–Gennaro, Lippincott William and Wilkins, New York, London – 2000, 1771.

203. *Ibid.*

204. Dr. Neelmani Ghatak. *Cause and Cure of Chronic Diseases*, Translator Chandra Shekhar Pathak. Publisher Dr. S.M. Bhattacharya, D.M.S. Kolkata F.P.T., Alipur, Kolkata - 700053, 4th edition, 81-82.

205. Dr. Neelmani Ghatak. *Cause and Cure of Chronic Diseases*, Translator Chandra Shekhar Pathak. Publisher Dr. S.M. Bhattacharya, D.M.S. Kolkata F.P.T., Alipur, Kolkata - 700053, 4th edition, 100-01, 152.

206. *Ibid.*

207. Dr. Neelmani Ghatak. *Cause and Cure of Chronic Diseases*, Translator Chandra Shekhar Pathak. Publisher Dr. S.M. Bhattacharya, D.M.S. Kolkata F.P.T., Alipur, Kolkata 700053, 4th edition, 223.

208. K. Park. *Park's Textbook of Preventive and Social Medicine,* 15th edition, Banarsidas Bhanot Publisher, Jabalpur, 1997, 91-100.

209. Samuel Hahnemann. *Organon of Medicine*, (English) Translated by William Boericke. B. Jain Publishers (P) Ltd., New Delhi - 110 055, 6th edition, 1993, pp. 36, 117.

210. Samuel Hahnemann, *Organon of Medicine,* (English) Translated by William Boericke. B. Jain Publishers (P) Ltd., New Delhi - 110 055, 6th edition, 1993, Paras 36-46, 117-32.

211. *Pathology,* edited by W.A.D. Anderson, 6th edition, Vol. 1, C.V. Mosby Company, 1971, 275.

212. Petersdorf, Adams, Braunwald. *Harrison's Principle of Internal Medicine,* 10th edition, McGraw Hill, 1983, New Delhi, 841.

213. David Greenwood, Richard Slack, *Medical – Microbiology*, 15th edition, Churchill Livingstone, New York, 1997.

214. David Greenwood, Richard Slack. *Medical – Microbiology*, 15th edition, Churchill Livingstone, New York, 1997, 149.

215. David Greenwood, Richard Slack. *Medical – Microbiology*, 15th edition, Churchill Livingstone, New York, 1997, 151.

216. David Greenwood, Richard Slack. *Medical – Microbiology*, 15th edition, Churchill Livingstone, New York, 1997, 152.

217. David Greenwood, Richard Slack. *Medical – Microbiology*, 15th edition, Churchill Livingstone, New York, 1997, 153.

218. *Pathology,* edited by W.A.D. Anderson, 6th edition, Vol. 1, C.V. Mosby Company, 1971, 378.

219. *Pathology,* edited by W.A.D. Anderson, 6th edition, Vol. 1, C.V. Mosby Company, 1971, 396.

220. *Pathology,* edited by W.A.D. Anderson, 6th edition, Vol. 1. C.V. Mosby Company, 1971, 394.

221. *Pathology,* edited by W.A.D. Anderson, 6th edition, Vol. 1. C.V. Mosby Company, 1971, 395.

222. *Op. cit.,* 220.

223. *Pathology,* edited by W.A.D. Anderson, 6th edition, Vol. 1, C.V. Mosby Company, 1971, 393.

224. K. Park. *Park's Textbook of Preventive and Social Medicine*, 15th edition, Banarsidas Bhanot Publisher, Jabalpur, 1997, 142.

225. K. Park. *Park's Textbook of Preventive and Social Medicine,* 15th edition. Banarsidas Bhanot Publisher, Jabalpur, 1997, 150.

226. Samuel Hahnemann. *Organon of Medicine* (English) Translated by William Boericke. B. Jain Publishers (P) Ltd., New Delhi - 110 055, 6th edition, 1993, Paras 46, 130.

227. W.A.D. Anderson. *Pathology*, Vol. 1, 6th edition, C.V. Mosby Company, St. Louis, 1971, 394.

228. Petersdorf, Adams, Braunwald. *Harrison's Principle of Internal Medicine,* 10th edition, McGraw Hill, 1983, New Delhi, 1190-95.

229. Samuel Hahnemann. *Organon of Medicine* (English) Translated by William Boericke. B. Jain Publishers (P) Ltd., New Delhi - 110 055, 6th edition, 1993, Paras 40, 125.

230. Satoskar, Bhandarkar. *Pharmacology & Pharmacotherapeutics.* Mumbai Popular Prakashan, 16th edition, 1999, 773-74.

231. Satoskar, Bhandarkar. *Pharmacology & Pharmacotherapeutics.* Mumbai Popular Prakashan, 16th edition, 1999, 774.

232. Craig and Stitzel. *Modern Pharmacology with Clinical Applications.* 5th edition, Little Brown and Company, New York, 1997, 611-612.

233. Goodman and Gilman's, *The Pharmacological Basis of Therapeutics*, 9th edition, McGraw Hill, New York, 1996, 1211.

234. James Tyler Kent, *Lectures on Homeopathic Philosophy.* B. Jain Publishers (P) Ltd., Delhi 1993, 52-53 (English language).

235. K. Park. *Park's Textbook of Preventive and Social Medicine* 15th edition, Banarsidas Bhanot Publishers, Jabalpur, 1997, 265.

236. John Macleod. *Davidson's Principles and Practice of Medicine.* 14th edition, E.L.B.S., Churchill Livingstone, 1984, 230-37.

237. Alfred Goodman Gilman, Louis Goodman, Alfred Gilman. *Goodman & Gilman's Prarmacological Basis of Therapeutics*, 6th edition, Macmillan 1980, 1080.

238. K. Park, *Park's Textbook of Preventive and Social Medicine,* 15th edition, Banarsidas Bhanot Publisher, Jabalpur, 1997, 265.

239. James Tyler Kent. *Lectures on Homeopathic Philosophy*. B. Jain Publishers (P) Ltd., Delhi 1993, 111 (English language).

240. James Tyler Kent. *Lectures on Homeopathic Philosophy*. B. Jain Publishers, Delhi, 1993, 11 (English language).

241. Petersdorf, Adams, Braunwald. *Harrison's Principle of Internal Medicine*, 10th edition, McGraw Hill, New Delhi, 1983, 675.

242. John Macleod. *Davidson's Principles and Practice of Medicine.* 14th edition, E.L.B.S., Churchill Livingstone, 1984, 462.

243. Petersdorf, Adams, Braunwald. *Harrison's Principle of Internal Medicine*, 10th edition, McGraw Hill, New Delhi, 1983, 677-78.

244. K. Park. *Park's Textbook of Preventive and Social Medicine,* 15th edition, Banarsidas Bhanot Publisher, Jabalpur, 1997, 150.

245. K. Park. *Park's Textbook of Preventive and Social Medicine,* 15th edition, Banarsidas Bhanot Publisher, Jabalpur, 1997, 26.

246. K. Park. *Park's Textbook of Preventive and Social Medicine,* 15th edition, Banarsidas Bhanot Publisher, Jabalpur, 1997, 84.

247. *Ibid.*

248. John, M. *A Dictionary of Epidemiology*. A handbook sponsored by the IEA, Oxford University Press, Last ed. (1983).

249. K. Park. *Park's Textbook of Preventive and Social Medicine,* 15th edition, Banarsidas Bhanot Publisher, Jabalpur, 1997, 88.

250. *Ibid.*

251. K. Park. *Park's Textbook of Preventive and Social Medicine,* 15th edition, Banarsidas Bhanot Publisher, Jabalpur, 1997, 88.

252. Rains and Ritchie. *Bailey & Love's Short Practice of Surgery,* 17th edition, H.K. Lewis & Co. 1977, 1073.

253. Petersdorf, Adams, Braunwald. *Harrison's Principle of Internal Medicine*, 10th edition, McGraw Hill, New Delhi, 1983, 959.

254. Petersdorf, Adams, Braunwald. *Harrison's Principle of Internal Medicine*, 10th edition, McGraw Hill, New Delhi, 1983, 675.

255. *Scientific American,* Aug. 1998 by Richard A. Deyo, 49-50.

256. J.R. Anderson. *Muir's Textbook of Pathology*. E.L.B.S., 12th edition, Edward Arnold London – introduction, 1985, 414.

257. IADVL. *Textbook of Skin Diseases*, Skin Disease by Pasricha, FITZPATRICK – Atlas of Skin Disease.

258. W.A.D. Anderson. *Pathology,* 6th edition, Vol. 1, C.V. Mosby Company, 1971, 286.

259. W.A.D. Anderson. *Pathology,* 6th edition, Vol. 1, C.V. Mosby Company, 1971, 551.

260. J.P. Brothers. *Ackarman's Surgical Pathology*, 7th edition, 1990, Delhi, Indian edition, 133.

261. J.R. Anderson. *Muir's Textbook of Pathology,* 10th edition, E.L.B.S., 12th edition, 1985, Edward Arnold London - introduction, 302.

262. Hellman Rosenberg. *Cancer,* edited by Devitta, 5th edition, Lippencott, Raven, New York, 1997, p. 966.

263. J.R. Anderson. *Muir's Textbook of Pathology*, 10th edition, E.L.B.S., 12th edition, 1985, Edward Arnold London - introduction, 307.

264. Katzung. *Basic and Clinical Pharmacology*, 4th edition, Lange Medical Book, Appleton & Lange Singapore, 1989.

265. Katzung. *Basic and Clinical Pharmacology*, 4th edition, Lange Medical Book, Appleton & Lange Singapore, 1989, 54.

266. Katzung. *Basic and Clinical Pharmacology*, 4th edition, Lange Medical Book, Appleton & Lange Singapore ,1989, 55.

267. Katzung. *Basic and Clinical Pharmacology*, 8th edition, Lange Medical Book, McGraw Hill, New York, 2001, 64.

268. Katzung. *Basic and Clinical Pharmacology*, 4th edition, Lange Medical Book, Appleton & Lange Singapore, 1989, 51.

269. Goodman and Gilman's. *The Pharmacological Basis of Therapeutics*, Vol.1, edition. McGraw Hill, New York, 1992, 76.

270. Katzung. *Basic and Clinical Pharmacology,* 4th edition, Lange Medical Book, Appleton & Lange, Sinapore, 1989, 56.

271. D.R. Laurence. *Clinical Pharmacoldogy*. E.B.S., 6th edition, 1987, 49.

272. Samuel Hahnemann. *Organon of Medicine* (English) Translated by William Boericke. B. Jain Publishers (P) Ltd., New Delhi - 110 055, 6th edition, 1993, 188. Samucl Hahnemann "Organon of Medicine" (Hindi) Translated by Prabha Devi. B. Jain Publishers, New Delhi, 1996, 120.

273. Samuel Hahnemann. *Organon of Medicine* (Hindi) Translated by Prabha Devi. B. Jain Publishers, New Delhi 1996, Paragraphs 107, 188.

274. Samuel Hahnemann. *Organon of Medicine* (Hindi) Translated by Prabha Devi. B. Jain Publishers, New Delhi, 1996, Paras 228, 120.

275. Samuel Hahnemann. *Organon of Medicine* (Hindi) Translated by Prabha Devi. B. Jain Publishers, New Delhi 1996, 52.

276. *Ibid.*

277. James Tyler Kent. *Lectures on Homeopathic Philosophy*. B. Jain Publishers (P) Ltd., New Delhi.

278. *Ibid.*

279. *Dorlands Medical Dictionary*. 24th edition, W.B. Saunders Company, London, 1965.

280. Petersdorf, Adams, Braunwald. *Harrison's Principle of Internal Medicine,* 10th edition, McGraw Hill, New Delhi, 1983, 1632.

281. Petersdorf, Adams, Braunwald. *Harrison's Principle of Internal Medicine,* 10th edition, McGraw Hill, New Delhi, 1983, 1633.

282. Petersdorf, Adams, Braunwald. *Harrison's Principle of Internal Medicine,* 10th edition, McGraw Hill, New Delhi, 1983, 1640.

283. Petersdorf, Adams, Braunwald. *Harrison's Principle of Internal Medicine,* 10th edition, McGraw Hill, New Delhi, 1983, 1635.

284. Petersdorf, Adams, Braunwald *Harrison's Principle of Internal Medicine,* 10th edition, McGraw Hill, New Delhi, 1983, 1038.

285. J.R. Anderson. *Muir's Textbook of Pathology*. 10th edition, E.L.B.S., 12th edition, 1976, 807.

286. Petersdorf, Adams, Braunwald.*Harrison's Principle of Internal Medicine*, 10th edition, McGraw Hill, New Delhi, 1983, 1036.

287. Petersdorf, Adams, Braunwald. *Harrison's Principle of Internal Medicine,* 10th edition, McGraw Hill, New Delhi, 1983, 1039.

288. James Tyler Kent. Kent *Lectures on Homeopathic Philosophy*. B. Jain Publishers (P) Ltd., Delhi, 1993, 63.

289. *Ibid.*

290. *Bally & Love's Short Practice of Surgery,* 17th edition, A.J. Harding Rains and H. David Ritchie London, H.K. Lewis & Co. Ltd., London 1977, 1078, 1081.

291. James Tyler Kent. *Lectures on Homeopathic Philosophy*. B. Jain Publishers (P) Ltd., Delhi, 1993, 186.

292. *Bally & Love's Short Practice of Surgery*, 17th edition, A.J. Harding Rains and H. David Ritchie London, H.K. Lewis & Co. Ltd., London 1977, 1080.

293. *Bally & Love's Short Practice of Surgery*, 17th edition, A.J. Harding Rains and H. David Ritchie London, H.K. Lewis & Co. Ltd., London 1977, 1078, 1081.

294. James Tyler Kent. *Lectures on Homeopathic Philosophy*. B. Jain Publishers (P) Ltd., Delhi, 1993, 54.

295. James Tyler Kent. *Lectures on Homeopathic Philosophy*. B. Jain Publishers (P) Ltd., Delhi, 1993, 55.

296. Kalpan and Sadock. *Comprehensive Textbook of Psychiarty*. 4th edition, Williams & Wilkins, USA, 1985, 838-45.

297. *Ibid.*

298. J.R. Anderson. *Muir's Textbook of Pathology*, 10th edition, E.L.B.S., London 12th edition, 1976, 538.

299. James Tyler Kent. *Lectures on Homeopathic Philosophy*. B. Jain Publishers (P) Ltd., Delhi, 1993, 34.

300. James Tyler Kent. *Lectures on Homeopathic Philosophy*. B. Jain Publishers (P) Ltd., Delhi, 1993, 44.

301. *Ibid.*
302. K. Park. *Park's Textbook of Preventive and Social Medicine.* 15th, edition, Banarsidas Bhanot Publisher, Jabalpur, 1997, 207-10.
303. Petersdorf, Adams, Braunwald. *Harrison's Principle of Internal Medicine.* 10th edition, McGraw Hill, New Delhi, 1983, 1136.
304. Samuel Hahnemann, *Organon of Medicine* (English) Translated by William Boericke. B. Jain Publishers (P) Ltd., New Delhi - 110 055, 6th edition, 1993, 44.
305. Samuel Hahnemann. *Organon of Medicine* (English) Translated by William Boericke. B. Jain Publishers (P) Ltd., New Delhi - 110 055, 6th edition, 1993, 22.
306. *Op. cit.,* 90.
307. Samuel Hahnemann. *Organon of Medicine* (English) Translated by William Boericke. B. Jain Publishers (P) Ltd., New Delhi - 110 055, 6th edition, 1993, 53.
308. *Op. cit.,* 90.
309. Petersdorf, Adams, Braunwald. *Harrison's Principle of Internal Medicine.* 10th edition, McGraw Hill, New Delhi, 1983, 932.
310. N.J. Modi. *Textbook of Medical Jurisprudence and Toxicology.* 9th edition, N.M. Tripathi Publisher Company, 1975, 631.
311. J.R. Anderson. *Muir's Text book of Pathology*, 10th edition, edited by E.L.B.S., Edward Arnold London, 170-71.
312. Guyton, John E. Hall. *Textbook of Medical Physiology*. Harcourt Asia Ltd., Singapore and W.B. Saunders Company, Philadelphia, 10th edition, 2000, 509.
313. Petersdorf, Adams, Braunwald. *Harrison's Principle of Internal Medicine*, 10th edition, McGraw Hill, New Delhi, 1983, 1009.
314. Samuel Hahnemann. *Organon of Medicine* (English) Translated by William Boericke. B. Jain Publishers (P) Ltd., New Delhi - 110 055, 6th edition, 1993, 45.
315. *Ibid.*
316. Philip Sartwell, edition, Maxcy Rosenau. *Preventive Medicine & Public Health*. (edited) 10th edition, Appleton – Century Crofts, New York 1973, 107.
317. Samuel Hahnemann. *Organon of Medicine* (English) Translated by William Boericke. B. Jain Publishers (P) Ltd., New Delhi - 110 055, 6th edition, 1993, 51.
318. *Op. cit.*, 90.
319. *Op. cit.*, 307.
320. Samuel Hahnemann. *Organon of Medicine* (English) Translated by William Boericke. B. Jain Publishers (P) Ltd., New Delhi - 110 055, 6th edition, 1993, 54.

321. Samuel Hahnemann. *Organon of Medicine* (English) Translated by William Boericke. B. Jain Publishers (P) Ltd., New Delhi - 110 055, 6th edition, 1993, 73.

322. *Ibid.*

323. Samuel Hahnemann. *Organon of Medicine* (English) Translated by William Boericke. B. Jain Publishers (P) Ltd., New Delhi - 110 055, 6th edition, 1993, 79.

324. Samuel Hahnemann. *Organon of Medicine* (English) Translated by William Boericke. B. Jain Publishers (P) Ltd., New Delhi - 110 055, 6th edition, 1993, Paras 72, 159.

325. *Op. cit.*, 90.

326. Samuel Hahnemann. *Organon of Medicine* (English) Translated by William Boericke. B. Jain Publishers (P) Ltd., New Delhi - 110 055, 6th edition, 1993, 52.

327. Samuel Hahnemann. *Organon of Medicine* (English) Translated by William Boericke. B. Jain Publishers (P) Ltd., New Delhi - 110 055, 6th edition, 1993, Paras 73, 160.

328. Samuel Hahnemann. *Organon of Medicine* (English) Translated by William Boericke. B. Jain Publishers (P) Ltd., New Delhi - 110 055, 6th edition, 1993, 69.

329. Samuel Hahnemann. *Organon of Medicine* (English) Translated by William Boericke. B. Jain Publishers (P) Ltd., New Delhi - 110 055, 6th edition, 1993, Paras 72, 159.

330. Samuel Hahnemann. *Organon of Medicine* (English) Translated by William Boericke. B. Jain Publishers (P) Ltd., New Delhi - 110 055, 6th edition, 1993, 9.

331. Samuel Hahnemann. *Organon of Medicine* (English) Translated by William Boericke. B. Jain Publishers (P) Ltd., New Delhi - 110 055, 6th edition, 1993, Paras 78, 166.

332. Samuel Hahnemann. *Organon of Medicine* (English) Translated by William Boericke. B. Jain Publishers (P) Ltd., New Delhi - 110 055, 6th edition, 1993, Paras 73, 160.

333. Samuel Hahnemann. *Organon of Medicine* (English) Translated by William Boericke. B. Jain Publishers (P) Ltd., New Delhi - 110 055, 6th edition, 1993, Paras 79, 166.

334. Petersdorf, Adams, Braunwald. *Harrison's Principle of Internal Medicine*, 10th edition, McGraw Hill, New Delhi, 1983, 1035.

335. John Macleod. *Davidson's Principles and Practice of Medicine*, 14th edition, E.L.B.S., Churchil Livingstone, 1984, 230-37.

336. E.C. Warner. *Savill's System of Clinical Medicine*, (edited), 14th edition, 1964, London Edward Arnold Publisher, 729.

337. Petersdorf, Adams, Braunwald. *Harrison's Principle of Internal Medicine*, 10th edition, McGraw Hill, 1983, New Delhi, 1035-36.

338. Petersdorf, Adams, Braunwald. *Harrison's Principle of Internal Medicine*, 10th edition, McGraw Hill, New Delhi, 1983, 1037.
339. Petersdorf, Adams, Braunwald. *Harrison's Principle of Internal Medicine*, 10th edition, McGraw Hill, New Delhi, 1983,1038.
340. Samuel Hahnemann. *The Chronic Diseases: Their Peculiar Nature and Their Homeopathic Cure*. Translated by Prof. Louish Tafel edited by Pemberton – Dudley. B. Jain Publilshers (P) Ltd., New Delhi, 1990, 87.
341. Samuel Hahnemann. *The Chronic Diseases: Their Peculiar Nature and Their Homeopathic Cure*. Translated by Prof. Louish Tafel edited by Pemberton – Dudley. B. Jain Publilshers (P) Ltd., New Delhi, 1990, 89.
342. Petersdorf, Adams, Braunwald. *Harrison's Principle of Internal Medicine*, 10th edition, McGraw Hill, 1983, New Delhi, 973-74.
343. Samuel Hahnemann. *The Chronic Diseases: Their Peculiar Nature and Their Homeopathic Cure*. Translated by Prof. Louish Tafel, edited Pemberton – Dudley. B. Jain Publilshers (P) Ltd., New Delhi, 1990, 88.
344. Maxcy Rosenau. *Preventive Medicine & Public Health,* edited by Philip Sartwell, 10th edition, Appleton Century Crofts, New York, 1973, 240-41.
345. E.C. Warner. *Savill's System of Clinical Medicine* (edited), 14th edition, 1964, London Edward Arnold Publisher, 731.
346. Frederick Forchheimer. *Therapeusis of Internal Diseases*, Vol. II, Butterworth, Sydney, London, 1913, 361-435.
347. *Ibid.*
348. Samuel Hahnemann. *The Chronic Diseases: Their Peculiar Nature and Their Homeopathic Cure*. Translated by Prof. Louish Tafel, edited by Pemberton – Dudley. B. Jain Publilshers (P) Ltd., New Delhi, 1990, 322.
349. Samuel Hahnemann. *Organon of Medicine*, (English) Translated by William Boericke. B. Jain Publishers (P) Ltd., New Delhi - 110 055, 6th edition, 1993, Paras 79, 294-95.
350. Samuel Hahnemann. *The Chronic Diseases: Their Peculiar Nature and their Homeopathic Cure*. Translated by Prof. Louish Tafel, edited Pemberton - Dudley. B. Jain Publilshers (P) Ltd., New Delhi, 1990, 150.
351. Samuel Hahnemann. *The Chronic Diseases: Their Peculiar Nature and Their Homeopathic Cure*. Translated by Prof. Louish Tafel, edited Pemberton - Dudley. B. Jain Publilshers (P) Ltd., New Delhi, 1990, 93.
352. Masters and Johnson. *Masters & Johnson on Sex & Human Loving*. Jaico Publishing House, Delhi, 1997, 535.
353. James Tyler Kent. *Lectures on Homeopathic Philosophy*. B. Jain Publishers (P) Ltd., Delhi, 1993, 142-43.
354. *Op. cit.,* 352.

355. Samuel Hahnemann. *The Chronic Diseases: Their Peculiar Nature and Their Homeopathic Cure*. Translated by Prof. Louish Tafel edited Pemberton – Dudley. B. Jain Publilshers (P) Ltd., New Delhi, 1990, 322.

356. *Ibid.*

357. James Crossland. *Lewis's Pharmacology*, 5th edition, Churchill Livingstone, New York 1980, 861-62.

358. E.C. Warner. *Savill's System of Clinical Medicine* (edited), 14th edition, 1964, London, Edward Arnold Publisher, 732.

359. Fitzpatrick, Eisen Wolff, Austen. *Dermatology in General Medicine*, 4th edition, Vol. II, McGraw Hill, New York, 1993, international edition, 2719.

360. James Tyler. *Lectures on Homeopathic Philosophy*. B. Jain Publishers (P) Ltd., Delhi, 1993, 141.

361. Petersdorf, Adams, Braunwald. *Harrison's Principle of Internal Medicine*, 10th edition, McGraw Hill, New Delhi, 1983, 1037.

362. James Tyler Kent. *Lectures on Homeopathic Philosophy*. B. Jain Publishers, Delhi, 1993, 142.

363. Petersdorf, Adams, Braunwald. *Harrison's Principle of Internal Medicine*, 10th edition, McGraw Hill, New Delhi, 1983, 974.

364. Samuel Hahnemann. *The Chronic Diseases* (Theoretical Part). B. Jain Publishers (P) Ltd., New Delhi, Reprint edition, 1999, 34-35.

365. Samuel Hahnemann. *The Chronic Diseases* (Theoretical Part). B. Jain Publishers (P) Ltd., New Delhi, Reprint edition, 1999, 34.

366. Samuel Hahnemann. *The Chronic Diseases* (Theoretical Part). B. Jain Publishers (P) Ltd., New Delhi, Reprint edition, 1999, 33.

367. Samuel Hahnemann. *The Chronic Diseases* (Theoretical Part). B. Jain Publishers (P) Ltd., New Delhi, Reprint edition, 1999, 40.

368. *Ibid.*

369. Samuel Hahnemann. *Organon of Medicine* (English) Translated by William Boericke. B. Jain Publishers (P) Ltd., New Delhi - 110 055, 6th edition, 1993, Paragraphs 79-80, 166-67.

370. Dr. Neelmani Ghatak. *Cause and Cure of Chronic Diseases*. Translator Chandra Shekhar Pathak. Publisher Dr. S.M. Bhattacharya, D.M.S. Kolkata F.P.T., Alipur, Kolkata - 700053, 4th edition, 241-42.

371. Dr. Neelmani Ghatak. *Cause and Cure of Chronic Diseases*. Translator Chandra Shekhar Pathak. Publisher Dr. S.M. Bhattacharya, D.M.S. Kolkata F.P.T., Alipur, Kolkata - 700053, 4th edition, 59-60.

372. Petersdorf, Adams, Braunwald. *Harrison's Principle of Internal Medicine*, 10th edition, McGraw Hill, New Delhi, 1983, 1000-01.

373. Samuel Hahnemann. *The Chronic Diseases* (Theoretical Part). B. Jain Publishers (P) Ltd., New Delhi, Reprint edition, 1999, 149-50.

374. Dr. Neelmani Ghatak. *Cause and Cure of Chronic Diseases* Translator Chandra Shekhar Pathak. Publisher Dr. S.M. Bhattacharya, D.M.S. Kolkata F.P.T., Alipur, Kolkata - 700053, 4th edition, 242.
375. Petersdorf, Adams, Braunwald. *Harrison's Principle of Internal Medicine*, 10th edition, McGraw Hill, 1983, New Delhi, 1000.
376. Petersdorf, Adams, Braunwald. *Harrison's Principle of Internal Medicine*, 10th edition, McGraw Hill, 1983, New Delhi, 1001.
377. Arthur Rook, D.S. Wilkinson, F.J.G. Ebling. *Textbook of Dermatology*, Vol. 1, 3rd edition, Blackwell Scientific Publication, Oxford London, 1979, 591.
378. K.M. Masani. *A Textbook of Gynaecology*, 7th edition, 1973, Popular Prakashan, Bombay, 304.
379. Maxcy Rosenau. *Preventive Medicine & Public Health*, edited by Philip Sartwe, 10th edition, Appleton Century Crofts, New York 1973, 242.
380. Petersdorf, Adams, Braunwald. *Harrison's Principle of Internal Medicine*, 10th edition, McGraw Hill, New Delhi, 1983, 1085.
381. Arthur Rook, D.S. Wilkinson, F.J.G. Ebling. *Textbook of Dermatology*, Vol. 1, 3rd edition, Blackwell Scientific Publication, Oxford London, 1979, 666.
382. Maxcy Rosenau. *Preventive Medicine & Public Health*, edited by Philip Sartwe, 10th edition, Appleton Century Crofts, New York, 1973, 240-41.
383. Fitzpatrick, Eisen Wolff, Austen. *Dermatology in General Medicine*, 4th edition, Vol. II, McGraw Hill, New York, 1993, international edition, 2752.
384. Eisen Wolff. *Dermatology in General Medicine*, 4th edition. editors Fitzpatrick, Austen, Vol. II, MacGraw Hill, New York, 1993, international edition, 1444.
385. *Ibid.*
386. Petersdorf, Adams, Braunwald. *Harrison's Principle of Internal Medicine*, 10th edition, McGraw Hill, 1983, New Delhi, 1174-75.
387. Fitzpatrick, Eisen Wolff, Austen. *Dermatology in General Medicine*, 4th edition, Vol. II, McGraw Hill, New York, 1993, international edition, 2619.
388. Arthur Rook, D.S. Wilkinson, F.J.G. Ebling. *Textbook of Dermatology*, Vol. 1, 3rd edition, Blackwell Scientific Publication, Oxford, London, 1979, 621.
389. Arthur Rook, D.S. Wilkinson, F.J.G. Ebling. *Textbook of Dermatology*. Vol.1, 3rd edition, Blackwell Scientific Publication, Oxford, London, 1979, 624.
390. *Ibid.*
391. Arthur Rook, D.S. Wilkinson, F.J.G. Ebling. *Textbook of Dermatology*, Vol. 1, 3rd edition, Blackwell Scientific Publication Oxford, London, 1979.

392. Rains and Ritchie. *Bailey & Love's Short Practice of Surgery*, 17th edition, H.K. Lewis & Co., 1977, 101.

393. Masters and Johnson. *Masters & Johnson on Sex & Human Loving*. Jaico Publishing House, Delhi, 1997, 536-43.

394. Petersdorf, Adams, Braunwald. *Harrison's Principle of Internal Medicine*, 10th edition, McGraw Hill, New Delhi, 1983, 940.

395. *Ibid.*

396. John Macleod. *Davidson's Principles and Practice of Medicine*, 14th edition, E.L.B.S., Churchill Livingstone, 1984, 411.

397. Petersdorf, Adams, Braunwald. *Harrison's Principle of Internal Medicine*, 10th edition, McGraw Hill, New Delhi, 1983, 941.

398. Rains and Ritchie. *Bailey & Love's Short Practice of Surgery*, 17th edition, H.K. Lewis & Co., 1977, 1067.

399. Fitzpatrick, Eisen Wolff, Austen. *Dermatology in General Medicine*, 4th edition, Vol. II, McGraw Hill, New York, 1993, international edition, 2611.

400. Samuel Hahnemann. *The Chronic Diseases* (Theoretical Part). B. Jain Publishers (P) Ltd., New Delhi, Reprint edition, 1999, 151.

401. Frederick Forchheimer. *Therapeutics of Internal Diseases*, Vol. II, Butterworth & Co., London and New York, 1913, 41.

402. Frederick Forchheimer. *Therapeutics of Internal Diseases*, Vol. II, Butterworth & Co., London and New York, 1913, 422.

403. Samuel Hahnemann. *The Chronic Diseases* (Theoretical Part). B. Jain Publishers (P) Ltd., New Delhi, Reprint edition, 1999, 155.

404. Samuel Hahnemann. *The Chronic Diseases* (Theoretical Part). B. Jain Publishers (P) Ltd., New Delhi, Reprint edition, 1999, 156.

405. Maxcy Rosenau. *Preventive Medicine & Public Health*, edited by Philip Sartwell, 10th edition, Appleton Century Crofts, New York 1973, 241.

406. Petersdorf, Adams Braunwald. *Harrison's Principle of Internal Medicine*, 10th edition, McGraw Hill, 1983, New Delhi, 374.

407. Samuel Hahnemann. *Organon of Medicine* (Hindi) Translator Prabha Devi (Prabhakar). B. Jain Publisher (P) Ltd., New Delhi 1996, 98.

408. Samuel Hahnemann. *Organon of Medicine* (Hindi) Translator Prabha Devi (Prabhakar). B. Jain Publisher (P) Ltd., New Delhi 1996, 100.

409. Samuel Hahnemann. *Organon of Medicine* (English) Translated by William Boericke. B. Jain Publishers (P) Ltd., New Delhi -110 055, 6th edition, 1993, 216.

410. Krantz and Carr. *The Pharmacological Principles of Medical Practice*, 6th edition, Williams and Wilkins Company, Baltimore 1965, 205-06.

411. David, Iswariah, Guruswami, *Pharmacology & Pharmacotherapeutics*, Revised by Iswariah and Guruswami. P. Vardacharya & Co., Madras, 1972, 7th edition, 626.

412. David, Iswariah, Guruswami. *Pharmacology & Pharmacotherapeutics*. Revised by Iswariah and Guruswami. P. Vardacharya & Co., Madras, 1972, 7th edition, 819.

413. David, Iswariah, Guruswami. *Pharmacology & Pharmacotherapeutics,* Revised by Iswariah and Guruswami. P. Vardacharya & Co., Madras, 1972, 7th edition, 740.

414. David, Iswariah, Guruswami. *Pharmacology & Pharmacotherapeutics,* Revised by Iswariah and Guruswami. P. Vardacharya & Co., Madras, 1972, 7th edition, 741-42.

415. David, Iswariah, Guruswami. *Pharmacology & Pharmacotherapeutics*. Revised by Iswariah and Guruswami. P. Vardacharya & Co., Madras, 1972, 7th edition, 748.

416. David, Iswariah, Guruswami. *Pharmacology & Pharmacotherapeutics,* Revised by Iswariah & Guruswami. P. Vardacharya & Co., Madras, 1972, 7th edition, 749.

417. Harry Beckman. *Treatment in General Practice*. 4th edition, W.B. Saunders Philadelphia1, 943, 719.

418. Dr. Neelmani Ghatak. *Cause and Cure of Chronic Diseases*, Translator Chandra Shekhar Pathak. Publisher Dr. S.M. Bhattacharya, D.M.S. Kolkata F.P.T., Alipur, Kolkata - 700053, 4th edition, 80-82.

419. James Tyler Kent. *Lectures on Homeopathic Philosophy*. B. Jain Publishers (P) Ltd., Delhi, 1993, 144.

420. King Nicole, Rodin. *Venereal Diseases*. ELBS and Bailliere Tindall, 4th edition, London, 1980, 363.

421. James Tyler Kent. *Lectures on Homeopathic Philosophy*. B. Jain Publishers (P) Ltd., Delhi, 1993, p. 146.

422. *Ibid.*

423. Petersdorf, Adams, Braunwald. *Harrison's Principle of Internal Medicine*. 10th edition, McGraw Hill, New Delhi, 1983, 941.

424. John Macleod. *Davidson's Principles and Practice of Medicine*. 14th edition, E.L.B.S., Churchill Livingstone, 1984, 411.

425. Fitzpatrick, Eisen Wolff, Austen. *Dermatology in General Medicine*, 4th edition, Vol. II, McGraw Hill, New York, 1993, international edition, 2611.

426. Beckman. *Pharmacology in Clinical Practice*. W.B. Saunders & Company, London, 1952, 708.

427. James Tyler Kent. *Lectures on Homeopathic Philosophy*. B. Jain Publishers (P) Ltd., Delhi, 1993, 146.

428. James Tyler Kent. *Lectures on Homeopathic Philosophy*. B. Jain Publishers (P) Ltd., Delhi, 1993, 146-47.

429. James Tyler Kent. *Lectures on Homeopathic Philosophy*. B. Jain Publishers (P) Ltd., Delhi, 1993, 147.

430. *Ibid.*

431. James Tyler Kent *Lectures on Homeopathic Philosophy*. B. Jain Publishers (P) Ltd., Delhi, 1993, 148.

432. *Ibid.*

433. A.J. Clark. *Applied Pharmacology*, 6th edition, London, J & A Churchill Ltd., 1938, 614.

434. A.J. Clark. *Applied Pharmacology*, 6th edition, London, J & A Churchill Ltd., 1938, 618.

435. A.J. Clark. *Applied Pharmacology*, 6th edition, London, J & A Churchill Ltd., 1938, 626-28.

436. A.J. Clark. *Applied Pharmacology*, 6th edition, London, J & A Churchill Ltd., 1938, 632.

437. Samuel Hahnemann. *The Chronic Diseases* (Theoretical Part). B. Jain Publishers (P) Ltd., New Delhi, Reprint edition, 1999, 15-19.

438. Krantz and Carr. *The Pharmacological Principles of Medical Practice*, 6th edition, Williams and Wilkins Company, Baltimore, 1965, 164.

439. Butter worth. *Therapeutics of Internal Diseases*, edited by Frederick Forchheimer, Vol. II, Sydney, London 1913, 406.

440. Alfred Goodman Gilman, Louis Goodman, Alfred Gilman. *Goodman & Gilman's Prarmacological Basis of Therapeutics*, 6th edition, Macmillan, 1980, 1631.

441. Gerstner, H. and Huff, J. *Clinical Toxicology of Mercury*. J. Toxicology, Environ. Health, 1977, 2, 491-526.

442. James Tyler Kent. *Lectures on Homeopathic Philosophy*. B. Jain Publishers (P) Ltd., Delhi, 1993, 147.

443. N.J. Modi. *Textbook of Medical Jurisprudence and Toxicology*, 9th edition, N.M. Tripathi Publisher Company, 1975, 526.

444. N.J. Modi. *Textbook of Medical Jurisprudence and Toxicology*. 9th edition, N.M. Tripathi Publisher Company, 1975, 529.

445. A.J. Clark. *Applied Pharmacology*, 6th edition, London, J & A Churchill Ltd., 1938, 632.

446. P.L. Soni. *Textbook of Inorganic Chemistry*. Sultan Publication, India, 2, 221.

447. James Tyler Kent. *Lectures on Homeopathic Philosophy*. B. Jain Publishers (P) Ltd., Delhi, 1993, 144-51.

448. N.J. Modi. *Textbook of Medical Jurisprudence and Toxicology*. 9th edition, N.M. Tripathi Publisher Company, 1975, 530.

449. N.J. Modi. *Textbook of Medical Jurisprudence and Toxicology*, 9th edition, N.M. Tripathi Publisher Company, 1975, 549-50.

450. *Op. cit.,* 445.

451. A.J. Clark. *Applied Pharmacology*, 6th edition, London, J & A Churchill Ltd., 1938, 620.

452. A.J. Clark. *Applied Pharmacology*, 6th edition, London. J & A Churchill Ltd., 1938, 623.

453. Frederick Forchheimer. *Therapeutics of Internal Diseases*, Vol. II, Butterworth & Co., London and New York, 1913, 383-84.
454. James Tyler Kent. *Lectures on Homeopathic Philosophy*. B. Jain Publishers (P) Ltd., Delhi, 1993, 143.
455. Samuel Hahnemann. *The Chronic Diseases* (Theoretical Part). B. Jain Publishers (P) Ltd., New Delhi, Reprint edition, 1999, 15-19.
456. James Tyler Kent. *Lectures on Homeopathic Philosophy*. B. Jain Publishers (P) Ltd., Delhi, 1993, 35.
457. James Tyler Kent. *Lectures on Homeopathic Philosophy*. B. Jain Publishers (P) Ltd., Delhi, 1993, 126.
458. James Tyler Kent. *Lectures on Homeopathic Philosophy*. B. Jain Publishers (P) Ltd., Delhi, 1993, 134.
459. James Tyler Kent. *Lectures on Homeopathic Philosophy*. B. Jain Publishers (P) Ltd., Delhi, 1993, 163.
460. Samuel Hahnemann. *The Chronic Diseases* (Theoretical Part). B. Jain Publishers (P) Ltd., New Delhi, Reprint edition, 1999, 163.
461. Samuel Hahnemann. *The Chronic Diseases* (Theoretical Part). B. Jain Publishers (P) Ltd., New Delhi, Reprint edition, 1999, 37.
462. Samuel Hahnemann. Reprint edition, 1999, 36.
463. James Tyler Kent. *Lectures on Homeopathic Philosophy*. B. Jain Publishers (P) Ltd., Delhi, 1993, 130.
464. James Tyler Kent. *Lectures on Homeopathic Philosophy*. B. Jain Publishers, Delhi, 1993, 135.
465. *Ibid.*
466. *Bible*. India Bible Literature Post Box 459, Madras, New Delhi, 1988, 4.
467. *Bible*. India Bible Literature Post Box 459, Madras, New Delhi, 1988, 73.
468. *Op. cit.*, 458.
469. *Bible*. India Bible Literature Post Box 459, Madras, New Delhi, 1988, 4.
470. Samuel Hahnemann. *The Chronic Diseases* (Theoretical Part). B. Jain Publishers (P) Ltd., New Delhi, Reprinit edition, 1999, 37.
471. James Crossland. *Lewis's Pharmacology*. 5th edition, Churchill Livingstone, New York, 1980, 294.
472. Petersdorf, Adams, Braunwald. *Harrison's Principle of Internal Medicine*. 10th edition, McGraw Hill, 1983, New Delhi, 1030.
473. Samuel Hahnemann. *The Chronic Diseases* (Theoretical Part). B. Jain Publishers (P) Ltd., New Delhi, Reprint edition, 1999, 38.
474. Petersdorf, Adams, Braunwald. *Harrison's Principle of Internal Medicine*. 10th edition, McGraw Hill, New Delhi, 1983, 1030.
475. W.A.D. Anderson. *Pathology*. Vol. 1, 6th edition, C.V. Mosby Company, St. Louis, 1971, 338.
476. Samuel Hahnemann. *The Chronic Diseases* (Theoretical Part). B. Jain Publishers (P) Ltd., New Delhi, Reprint edition, 1999, 37.

477. Samuel Hahnemann. *The Chronic Diseases* (Theoretical Part). B. Jain Publishers (P) Ltd., New Delhi, Reprint edition, 1999, 41.
478. Samuel Hahnemann. *The Chronic Diseases* (Theoretical Part). B. Jain Publishers (P) Ltd., New Delhi, Reprint edition, 1999, 42-43.
479. Samuel Hahnemann. *The Chronic Diseases* (Theoretical Part). B. Jain Publishers (P) Ltd., New Delhi, Reprint edition, 1999, 42.
480. Samuel Hahnemann. *The Chronic Diseases* (Theoretical Part). B. Jain Publishers (P) Ltd., New Delhi, Reprint edition, 1999, 105-43.
481. Samuel Hahnemann. *The Chronic Diseases* (Theoretical Part). B. Jain Publishers (P) Ltd., New Delhi, Reprint edition, 1999, 143.
482. Samuel Hahnemann. *The Chronic Diseases* (Theoretical Part). B. Jain Publishers (P) Ltd., New Delhi, Reprint edition, 1999, 78-79.
483. Samuel Hahnemann. *The Chronic Diseases* (Theoretical Part). B. Jain Publishers (P) Ltd., New Delhi, Reprint edition, 1999, 80.
484. Samuel Hahnemann. *The Chronic Diseases* (Theoretical Part). B. Jain Publishers (P) Ltd., New Delhi, Reprint edition, 1999, 81.
485. Samuel Hahnemann. *The Chronic Diseases* (Theoretical Part). B. Jain Publishers (P) Ltd., New Delhi, Reprint edition, 1999, 87.
486. Samuel Hahnemann. *The Chronic Diseases* (Theoretical Part). B. Jain Publishers (P) Ltd., New Delhi, Reprint edition, 1999, 98.
487. *Op. cit.,* 477.
488. Samuel Hahnemann. *The Chronic Diseases* (Theoretical Part). B. Jain Publishers (P) Ltd., New Delhi, Reprint edition, 1999, 48.
489. *Ibid.*
490. Samuel Hahnemann. *The Chronic Diseases* (Theoretical Part). B. Jain Publishers (P) Ltd., New Delhi, Reprint edition, 1999, 35.
491. Samuel Hahnemann. *The Chronic Diseases* (Theoretical Part). B. Jain Publishers (P) Ltd., New Delhi, Reprint edition, 1999, 41.
492. Samuel Hahnemann. *The Chronic Diseases* (Theoretical Part). B. Jain Publishers (P) Ltd., New Delhi, Reprint edition, 1999, 62.
493. Samuel Hahnemann. *The Chronic Diseases* (Theoretical Part). B. Jain Publishers (P) Ltd., New Delhi, Reprint edition, 1999, 51.
494. Petersdorf, Adams, Braunwald, *Harrison's Principle of Internal Medicine*, 10th edition, McGraw Hill, New Delhi, 1983, 1065.
495. Samuel Hahnemann. *The Chronic Diseases* (Theoretical Part). B. Jain Publishers (P) Ltd., New Delhi, Reprint edition, 1999, 49-69.
496. Petersdorf, Adams, Braunwald. *Harrison's Principle of Internal Medicine*, 10th edition, McGraw Hill, New Delhi, 1983, 1512.
497. Petersdorf, Adams, Braunwald. *Harrison's Principle of Internal Medicine*, 10th (edition) McGraw Hill, New Delhi, 1983, 1512-19.
498. E.C. Warner. *Savill's System of Clinical Medicine* (edited), 14th edition. 1964, London Edward Arnold Publisher, 211.

499. E.C. Warner. *Savill's System of Clinical Medicine* (edited), 14th edition, 1964, London Edward Arnold Publisher, 214.
500. Samuel Hahnemann. *The Chronic Diseases* (Theoretical Part). B. Jain Publishers (P) Ltd., New Delhi, Reprint edition, 1999, 64.
501. Samuel Hahnemann. *The Chronic Diseases* (Theoretical Part). B. Jain Publishers (P) Ltd., New Delhi, Reprint edition, 1999, 66.
502. *Ibid.*
503. Samuel Hahnemann. *The Chronic Diseases* (Theoretical Part). B. Jain Publishers (P) Ltd., New Delhi, Reprint edition, 1999, 67.
504. Petersdorf, Adams, Braunwald. *Harrison's Principle of Internal Medicine*, 10th edition, McGraw Hill, 1983, New Delhi, 2018-27.
505. E.C. Warner. *Savill's System of Clinical Medicine* edited, 14th edition, 1964, London Edward Arnold Publisher, 1141.
506. *Ibid.*
507. Samuel Hahnemann *The Chronic Diseases* (Theoretical Part). B. Jain Publishers (P) Ltd., New Delhi, Reprint edition, 1999, 63.
508. Petersdorf, Adams, Braunwald. *Harrison's Principle of Internal Medicine*, 10th edition, McGraw Hill, 1983, New Delhi, 1110.
509. Petersdorf, Adams, Braunwald. *Harrison's Principle of Internal Medicine*, 10th edition, McGraw Hill, 1983, New Delhi, 1109.
510. Petersdorf, Adams, Braunwald. *Harrison's Principle of Internal Medicine*, 10th edition, McGraw Hill, 1983, New Delhi, 1109-11.
511. E.C. Warner. *Savill's System of Clinical Medicine* (edited) 14th edition, 1964, London Edward Arnold Publisher, 669.
512. E.C. Warner. *Savill's System of Clinical Medicine* (edited) 14th edition, 1964, London Edward Arnold Publisher, 670.
513. E.C. Warner. *Savill's System of Clinical Medicine* (edited) 14th edition, 1964, London Edward Arnold Publisher, 673-74.
514. E.C. Warner. *Savill's System of Clinical Medicine* (edited) 14th edition, 1964, London Edward Arnold Publisher, 678.
515. E.C. Warner. *Savill's System of Clinical Medicine* (edited) 14th edition, 1964, London Edward Arnold Publisher, 695.
516. E.C. Warner. *Savill's System of Clinical Medicine* edited, 14th edition, 1964, London Edward Arnold Publisher, 702.
517. E.C. Warner. *Savill's System of Clinical Medicine* (edited) 14th edition, 1964, London Edward Arnold Publisher, 709.
518. Samuel Hahnemann. *The Chronic Diseases* (Theoretical Part). B. Jain Publishers (P) Ltd., New Delhi, Reprint edition, 1992, 62.
519. *Ibid.*
520. Samuel Hahnemann. *The Chronic Diseases* (Theoretical Part). B. Jain Publishers (P) Ltd., New Delhi, Reprint edition, 1992, 65.
521. *Op. cit.*, 519.

522. Samuel Hahnemann. *The Chronic Diseases* (Theoretical Part). B. Jain Publishers (P) Ltd., New Delhi, Reprint edition, 1992, 169-74.

523. Samuel Hahnemann. *The Chronic Diseases* (Theoretical Part). B. Jain Publishers (P) Ltd., New Delhi, Reprint edition, 1992, 51-69.

524. Samuel Hahnemann. *Organon of Medicine* (English) Translated by William Boericke. B. Jain Publishers (P) Ltd., New Delhi - 110 055, 6th edition, 1993, Paragraphs 154, 218.

525. Samuel Hahnemann. *Organon of Medicine* (English) Translated by William Boericke. B. Jain Publishers (P) Ltd., New Delhi - 110 055, 6th edition, 1993, Paragraphs 246, 270.

526. Samuel Hahnemann. *Organon of Medicine* (English) Translated by William Boericke. B. Jain Publishers (P) Ltd., New Delhi - 110 055, 6th edition, 1993, Paragraphs 247, 272.

527. Samuel Hahnemann. *The Chronic Diseases* (Theoretical Part). B. Jain Publishers (P) Ltd., New Delhi, Reprint edition, 1999, 212.

528. Samuel Hahnemann. *Organon of Medicine* (English) Translated by William Boericke. B. Jain Publishers (P) Ltd., New Delhi - 110 055, 6th edition, 1993, Paragraphs 247, 272.

529. Samuel Hahnemann. *The Chronic Diseases* (Theoretical Part). B. Jain Publishers (P) Ltd., New Delhi, Reprint edition, 1999, 214.

530. Samuel Hahnemann. *The Chronic Diseases* (Theoretical Part). B. Jain Publishers (P) Ltd., New Delhi, Reprint edition, 1999, 215.

531. Samuel Hahnemann. *The Chronic Diseases* (Theoretical Part). B. Jain Publishers (P) Ltd., New Delhi, Reprint edition, 1999, 216.

532. Samuel Hahnemann. *The Chronic Diseases* (Theoretical Part). B. Jain Publishers (P) Ltd., New Delhi, Reprint edition, 1999, 216-17.

533. Samuel Hahnemann. *The Chronic Diseases* (English) Translated by William Boericke. B. Jain Publishers (P) Ltd., New Delhi - 110 055, 6th edition, 1993, Paragraphs 248, 275.

534. Samuel Hahnemann. *The Chronic Diseases* (Theoretical Part). B. Jain Publishers (P) Ltd., New Delhi, Reprint edition, 1999, 220.

535. Samuel Hahnemann. *The Chronic Diseases* (Theoretical Part). B. Jain Publishers (P) Ltd., New Delhi, Reprint edition, 1999, 219-20.

536. Samuel Hahnemann. *Organon of Medicine* (English) Translated by William Boericke. B. Jain Publishers (P) Ltd., New Delhi - 110 055, 6th edition, 1993, 306.

537. K. Park. *Park's Textbook of Preventive and Social Medicine*, 15th edition, Banarsidas Bhanot Publisher, Jabalpur, 1997, 174.

538. K. Park. *Park's Textbook of Preventive and Social Medicine*, 15th edition Banarsidas. Bhanot Publisher, Jabalpur, 1997, 50.

539. K. Park. *Park's Textbook of Preventive and Social Medicine*. 15th edition Banarsidas Bhanot Publisher, Jabalpur, 1997, 118.

540. E.C. Warner. *Savill's System of Clinical Medicine,* 14th edition, 1964, London Edward Arnold Publisher, 712.

541. K. Park. *Park's Textbook of Preventive and Social Medicine*, 15th edition, Banarsidas Bhanot Publisher, Jabalpur, 1997, 158.
542. K. Park. *Park's Text Book of Preventive and Social Medicine*, 15th edition, Banarsidas, Bhanot Publisher, Jabalpur, 1997, 159.
543. E.C. Warner. *Savill's System of Clinical Medicine* (edited), 14th edition, 1964, London Edward Arnold Publisher, 195-96.
544. D.R. Laurance. *Clinical Pharmacology*, P.N. Bennet, 7th edition, E.L.B.S., Churchill Livingstone, 1992, 19-20.
545. Samuel Hahnemann. *The Chronic Diseases* (Theoretical Part). B. Jain Publishers (P) Ltd., New Delhi, Reprint edition, 1992, 174.
546. Samuel Hahnemann. *The Chronic Diseases* (Theoretical Part). B. Jain Publishers (P) Ltd., New Delhi, Reprint edition, 1992, 203.
547. Samuel Hahnemann. *The Chronic Diseases* (Theoretical Part). B. Jain Publishers (P) Ltd., New Delhi, Reprint edition, 1992, 193.
548. *Ibid.*
549. *Ibid.*
550. Samuel Hahnemann. *The Chronic Diseases* (Theoretical Part). B. Jain Publishers (P) Ltd., New Delhi, Reprint edition, 1992, 193-94.
551. Samuel Hahnemann. *The Chronic Diseases* (Theoretical Part). B. Jain Publishers (P) Ltd., New Delhi, Reprint edition, 1992, 194.
552. *Ibid.*
553. Samuel Hahnemann. *The Chronic Diseases* (Theoretical Part). B. Jain Publishers (P) Ltd., New Delhi, Reprint edition, 1992, 195.
554. Samuel Hahnemann. *The Chronic Diseases* (Theoretical Part). B. Jain Publishers (P) Ltd., New Delhi, Reprint edition, 1992, 195-96.
555. Samuel Hahnemann. *The Chronic Diseases* (Theoretical Part). B. Jain Publishers (P) Ltd., New Delhi, Reprint edition, 1992, 200.
556. Samuel Hahnemann. *The Chronic Diseases* (Theoretical Part). B. Jain Publishers (P) Ltd., New Delhi, Reprint edition, 1992, 201.
557. *Ibid.*
558. Samuel Hahnemann. *The Chronic Diseases* (Theoretical Part). B. Jain Publishers (P) Ltd., New Delhi, Reprint edition, 1992, 209.
559. Samuel Hahnemann. *The Chronic Diseases* (Theoretical Part). B. Jain Publishers (P) Ltd., New Delhi, Reprint edition, 1992, 213.
560. Samuel Hahnemann. *The Chronic Diseases* (Theoretical Part). B. Jain Publishers (P) Ltd., New Delhi, Reprint edition, 1992, 215.
561. Samuel Hahnemann. *The Chronic Diseases* (Theoretical Part). B. Jain Publishers (P) Ltd., New Delhi, Reprint edition, 1992, 224-25.
562. Samuel Hahnemann. *The Chronic Diseases* (English) Translated by William Boericke. B. Jain Publilshers (P) Ltd., New Delhi - 110 055, 6th edition, 1993, Paragraphs 276, 299.
563. Samuel Hahnemann. *The Chronic Diseases* (Theoretical Part). B. Jain Publishers (P) Ltd., New Delhi, Reprint edition, 1992, Paragraphs 260, 281.

564. Samuel Hahnemann *The Chronic Diseases* (Theoretical Part). B. Jain Publishers (P) Ltd., New Delhi, Reprint edition, 1992, 281-82.

565. Samuel Hahnemann. *The Chronic Diseases* (Theoretical Part). B. Jain Publishers (P) Ltd., New Delhi, Reprint edition, 1999, 335.

566. Petersdorf, Adams, Braunwald Harrison's. *Principles of Internal Medicine*, 10th edition, McGraw Hill, 1983, New Delhi, 1120.

567. Petersdorf, Adams, Braunwald Harrison's. *Principles of Internal Medicine*, 10th edition, McGraw Hill, 1983, New Delhi, 961.

568. John Macleod. *Davidson's Principles and Practice of Medicine*. 14th edition.0 E.L.B.S., Churchill Livingstone, London 1984, 230-37.

569. John Macleod *Davidson's. Principles and Practice of Medicine.* 14th edition, E.L.B.S., Churchill Livingstone, 1984, 748.

570. Samuel Hahnemann. *The Chronic Diseases* (Theoretical Part). B. Jain Publishers (P) Ltd., New Delhi, Reprint edition, 1999, 228.

571. Samuel Hahnemann. *The Chronic Diseases* (Theoretical Part), B. Jain Publishers (P) Ltd., New Delhi, Reprint edition, 1999, 233.

572. Rang, Dale, Ritter, Moore. *Pharmacology*. 5th edition, Churchill Livingstone, New York, 2003, 3-4.

573. Laurance, Bennet, Brown. *Clinical Pharmacology*. 8th edition, Churchill Livingstone, New York, 1997, 13-14.

574. *Op. cit.,* 5.

575. Satoskar and Bhandarkar. *Pharmacology & Pharmacotherapeutics*. 18th edition, Popular Prakashan, Mumbai, 2003, 2.

576. *The Hindu*. Delhi 27th August 2005, p. 20.

BIBLIOGRAPHY

Abnormal Psychology and Modern Life, James Coleman

The Science and Practice of Pharmacy, Remington

Clinical Pharmacology, D.R. Laurence

Applied Pharmacology by Models, Schield

The Pharmacological Basis of Medical Practice, Krants and Carr

Dril's Pharmacology in Medicine, Dipolmo, Joseph

French's Index of Differential Diagnosis, F. Dudley Hart

Harrison's Principle of Internal Medicine, Petersdorf, Adams

Pharmacology and Pharmacotherapeutics, Satoskar, Bhandarkar

Goodman and Gilma's Pharmacological Basis of therapeutics, Goodman, Gilman

Text book of Medical Jurisprudence and Toxicology, N.J. Modi

Modern Pharmacology, Craig and Stitzel

Organon of Medicine, Samuel Hahnemann

Lectures on Homeopathic Philosophy, James Kent.

Muir's Text book of Pathology, J.R. Anderson

Park's Text Book of Preventive and Social Medicine, K. Park

Pathology, W.A.D. Anderson

Review of Medical Physiology, William Ganong

A Text Book of Medical Physiology, Guyton and Hall

Life of Christian Samuel Hahnemann, Rosa Waugh Bobhouse

Text Book of Psychiatry, Talbott, Hales

Price's Text Book of Practice of Medicine, Ronald Bodley

Bailey and Love's Short Practice of Surgery, Rains and Ritchie

Text Book of Inorganic Chemistry, P.L. Soni

Text Book of Physical Chemistry, P.L. Soni

Cause and Cure of Chronic Diseases a Homeopathic book, Dr. Neelmani Ghatak

Comprehensive Text Book of Psychiatry, Kaplan and Sadock. *Medical Microbiology* by David Grenwood, Richard Slack

Davidson's Principles and Practice of Medicine, John Macleod

A Dictionary of Epidemiology, Oxford University Press

Text Book of Skin Disease?

Ackarman's Surgical Pathology by J.P. Brothers

Cancer, Devitta, Hellman Rosenberg

Basic and Clinical Pharmacology by Katzung

Dorlands Medical Dictionary

Kent Lecture on Homeopathic Philosophy by James Tayler Kent

Preventive Medicine and Public Health by Maxcy Rosenau

The Chronic Disease, their peculiar nature and their homeopathic cure by Samuel Hahnemann.

Savill's System of Clinical Medicine by E.C. Warner

Therapeusis of Internal Diseases, Frederick Forchheimer

Masters and Johnson on Sex and Human Loving, Masters and Johnson

Lewi's Pharmacology, James Crossland

Dermatology in General Medicine, Fitzpatrick, Wolff

The Chronic Diseases (Theoretical Part), Samuel Hahnemann

Text Book of Dermatology, Arthur Rook, Wilkinson

A Text book of Gynaecology, K.M. Masani

Pharmacology and Pharmacotherapeutics, David, Iswarias

Treatment in General Practice Harry Beckman

Venereal Diseases, King Nicol

Pharmacology in Clinical Practice, Becknman

Applied Pharmacology, A.J. Clark

Clinical Toxicology on Mercury, Gerstner and Huff

The Bible